Dedicated to nurses and nursing students worldwide.
Being a nurse is a precious gift, cherish it.

Don't be a nurse they said,
And with that I simply hung my head.

Being a nurse is more than bedpans and call lights, It's
fighting for every single patient's rights.

I am a nurse because it's my call.
Something I've felt since I was small.

If you have a minute, I'll tell you why I became a nurse,
at least I'll try.

So, what does being a nurse mean to me?
I'll give you 26 reasons from A-to-Z.

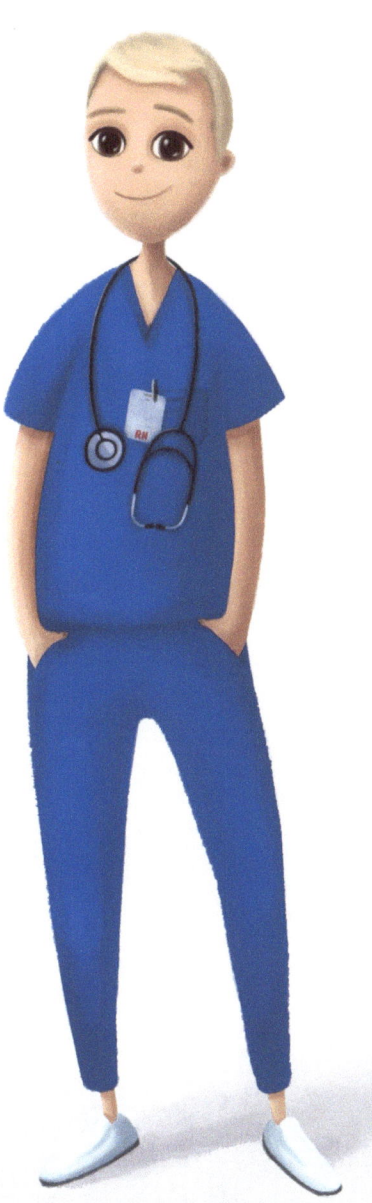

A is for Advocate

A nurse always ensures the best for their patient. The nurse defends, supports, and acts as a liaison between the patient and the provider ensuring patients before profits.

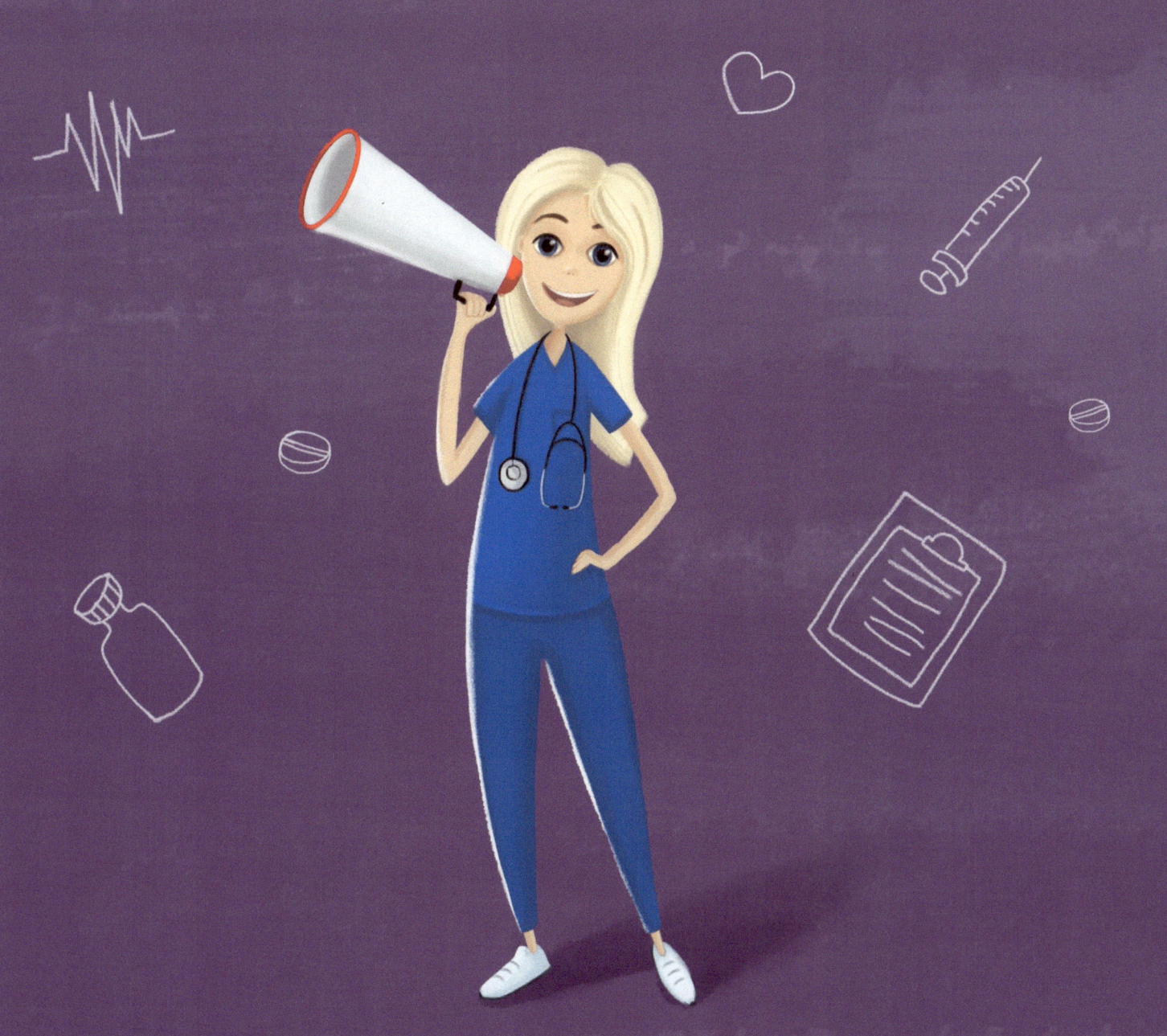

B is for Benevolent

In every action the nurse is kind and well meaning. Others above self. Shift after shift, the nurse puts themselves into danger. Danger of infection, danger of death, danger of litigation, danger. This does not deter the nurse who means well and is kind to all.

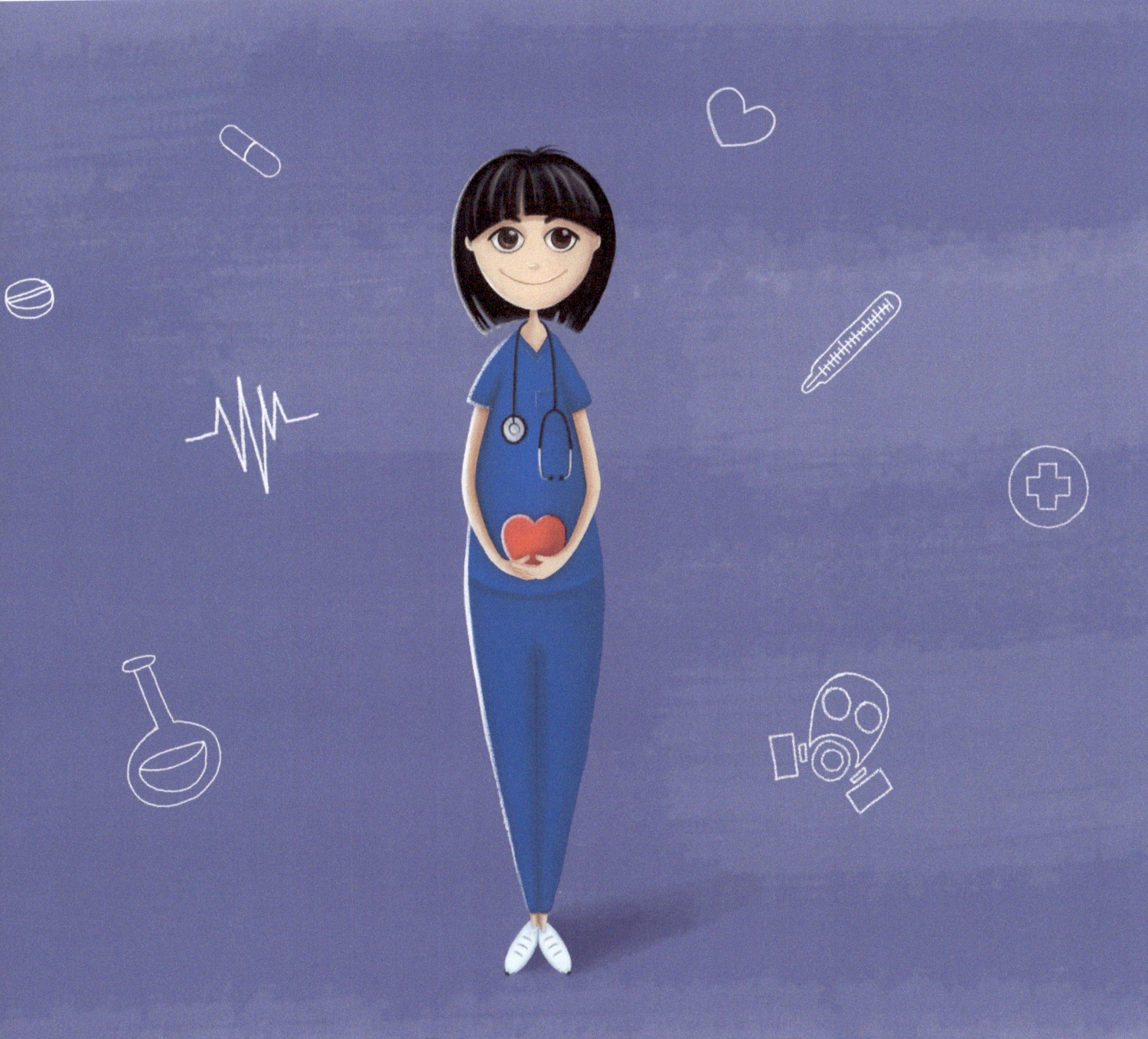

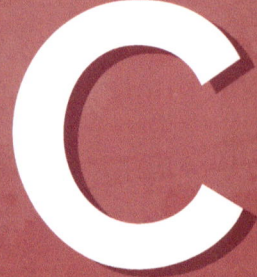

C is for Calming

Despite the craziness of the situation, the nurse brings calm. Just the presence of a nurse can calm the dying patient, comfort the scared infant, or calm the nervous family.

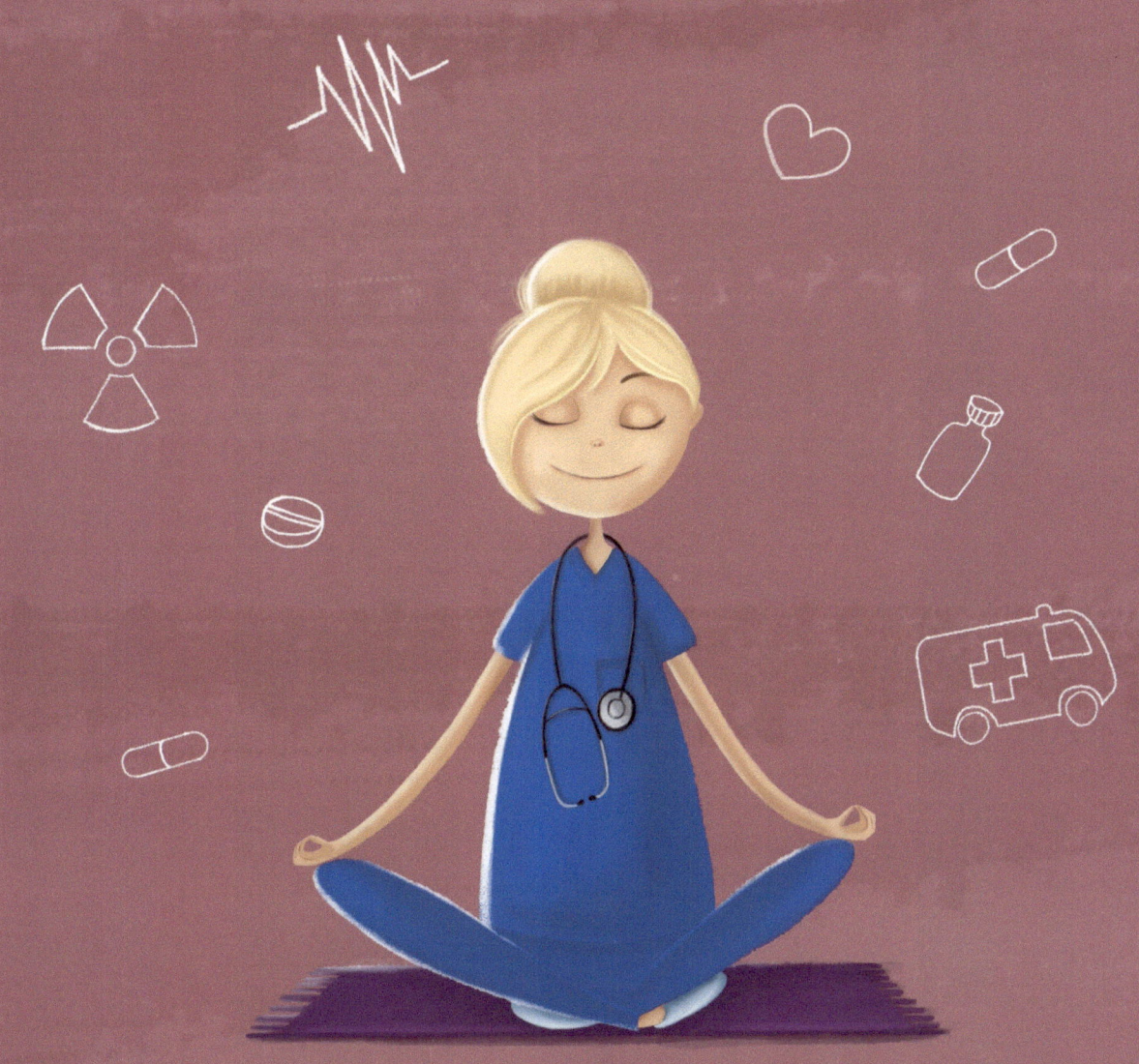

D
is for Dedication

No other job demands so much emotion, hard work, and dedication as nursing. The nurse knows this. In the midst of a 14 hour shift, with little sleep, no food, dealing with life and death, the nurse remains dedicated to caring for the patient.

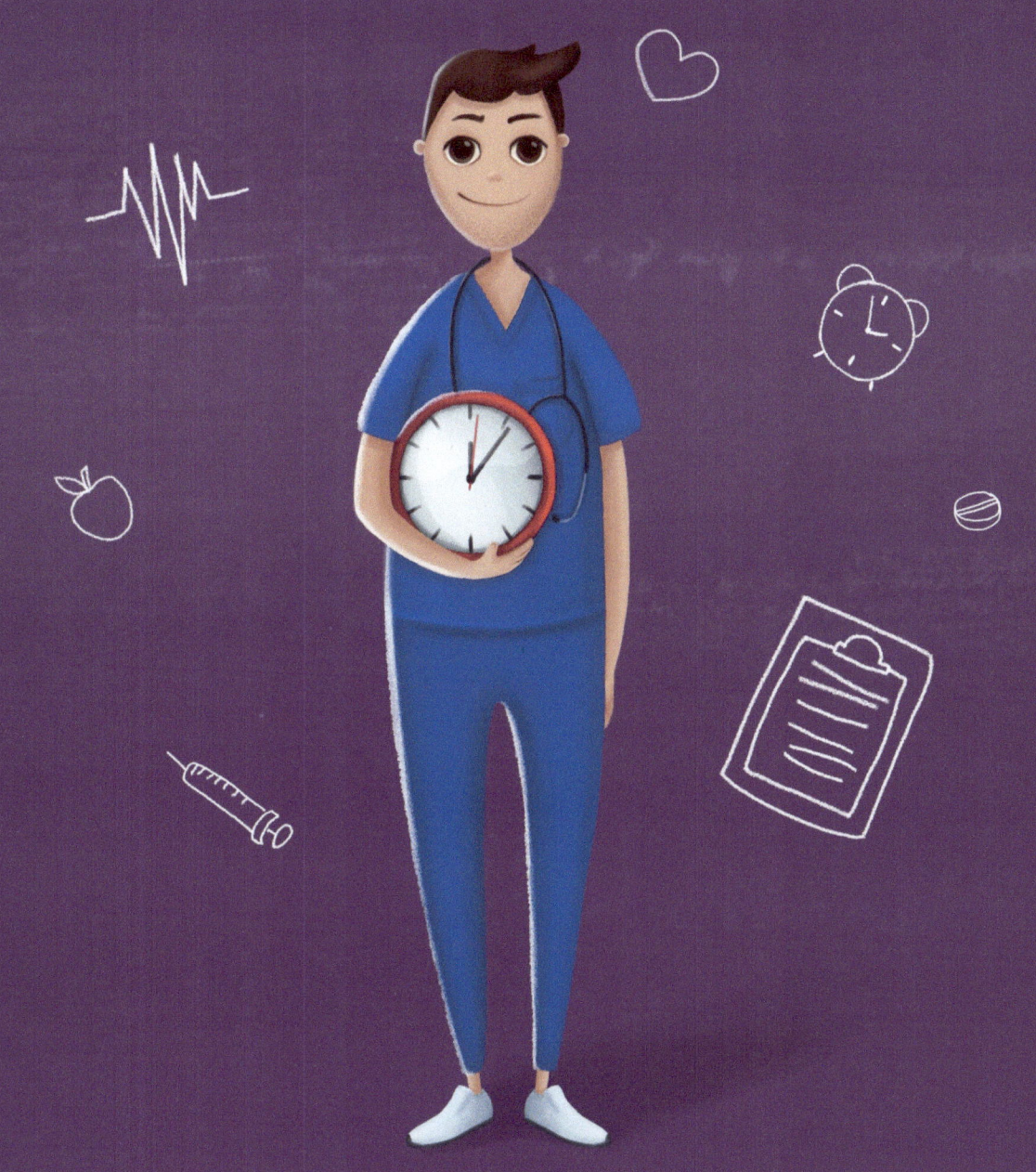

E

is for Empathy

The nurse will sit in a room with a family and patient after hearing devastating news. The nurse will feel their pain, cry with them, share with them, and give of self with no thought of their own needs.

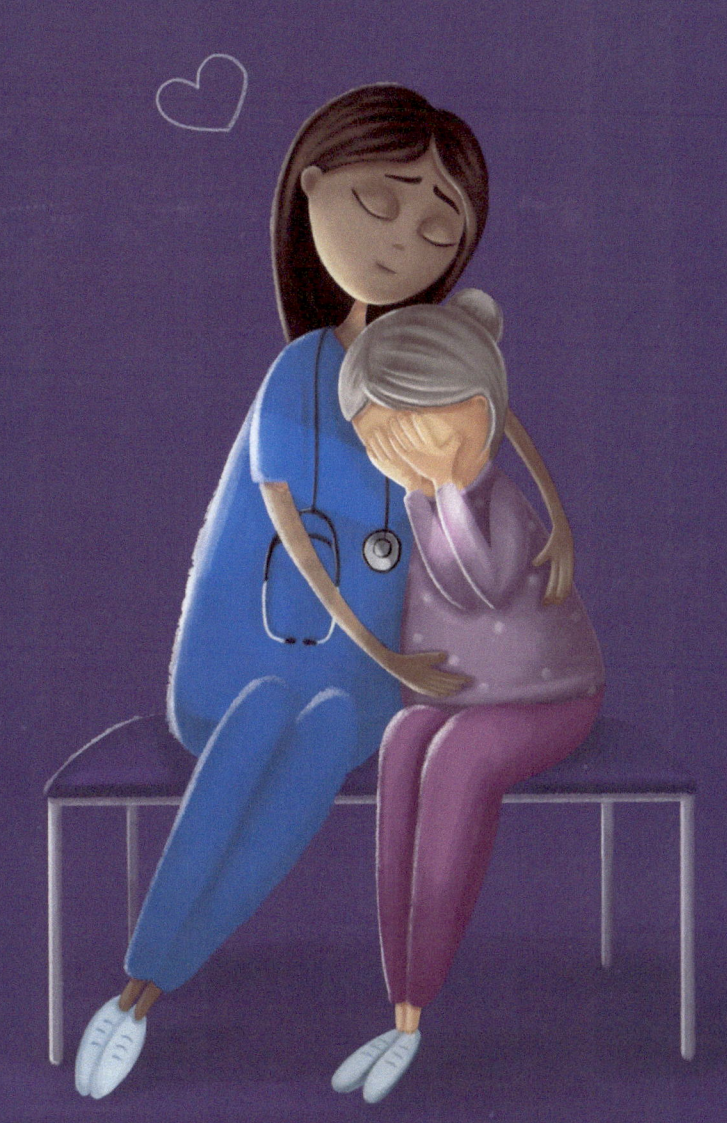

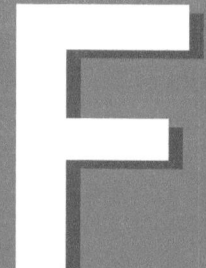

F

is for Friendly

Despite the stress, the nurse will smile and share with each new patient. The nurse understands that a smile and a gentle touch can calm the storm inside a nervous patient.

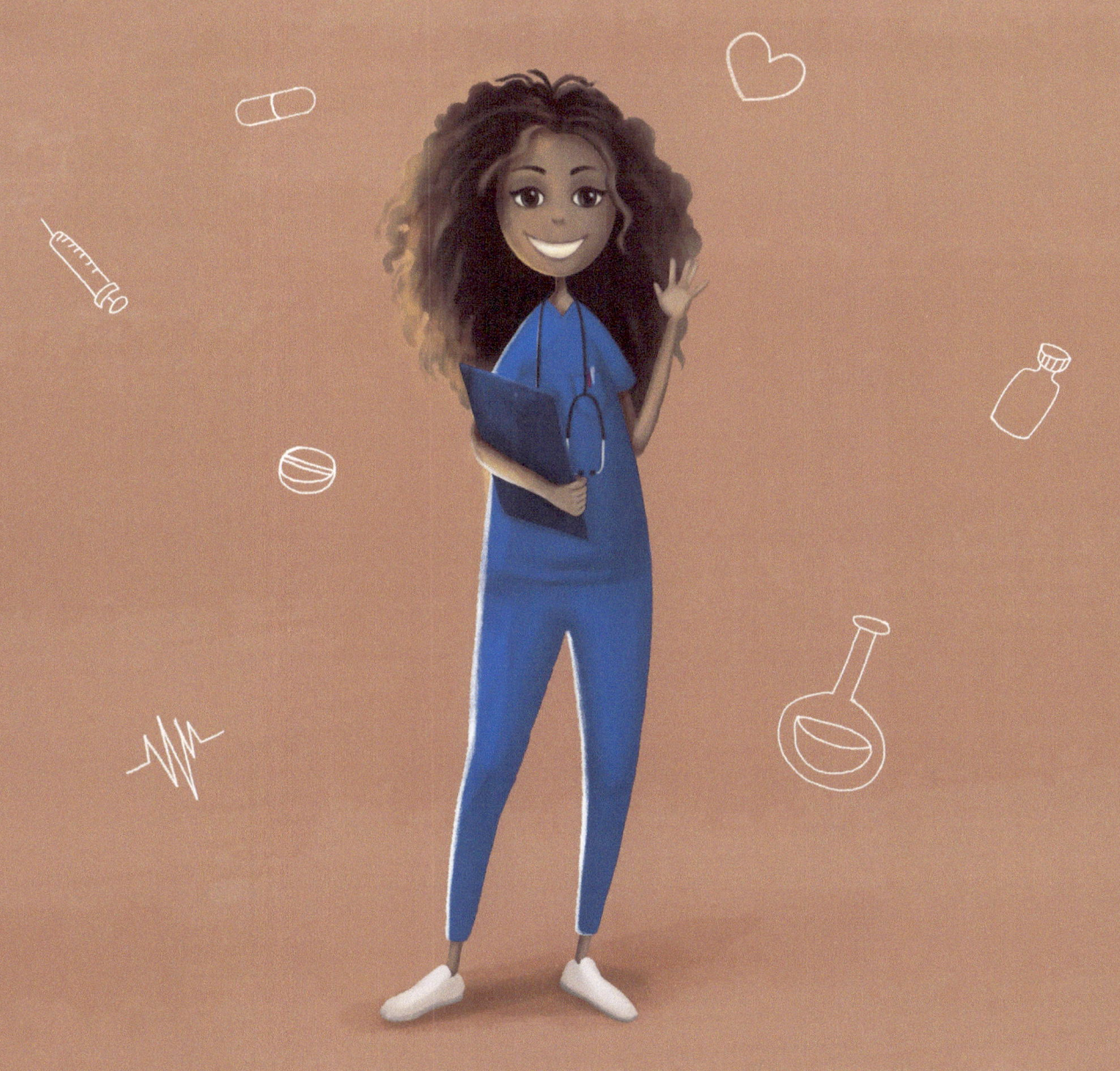

G is for Guardian

Patients put their trust in the nurse to protect and guard them through the entire healthcare process. The nurse keeps the patient safe.

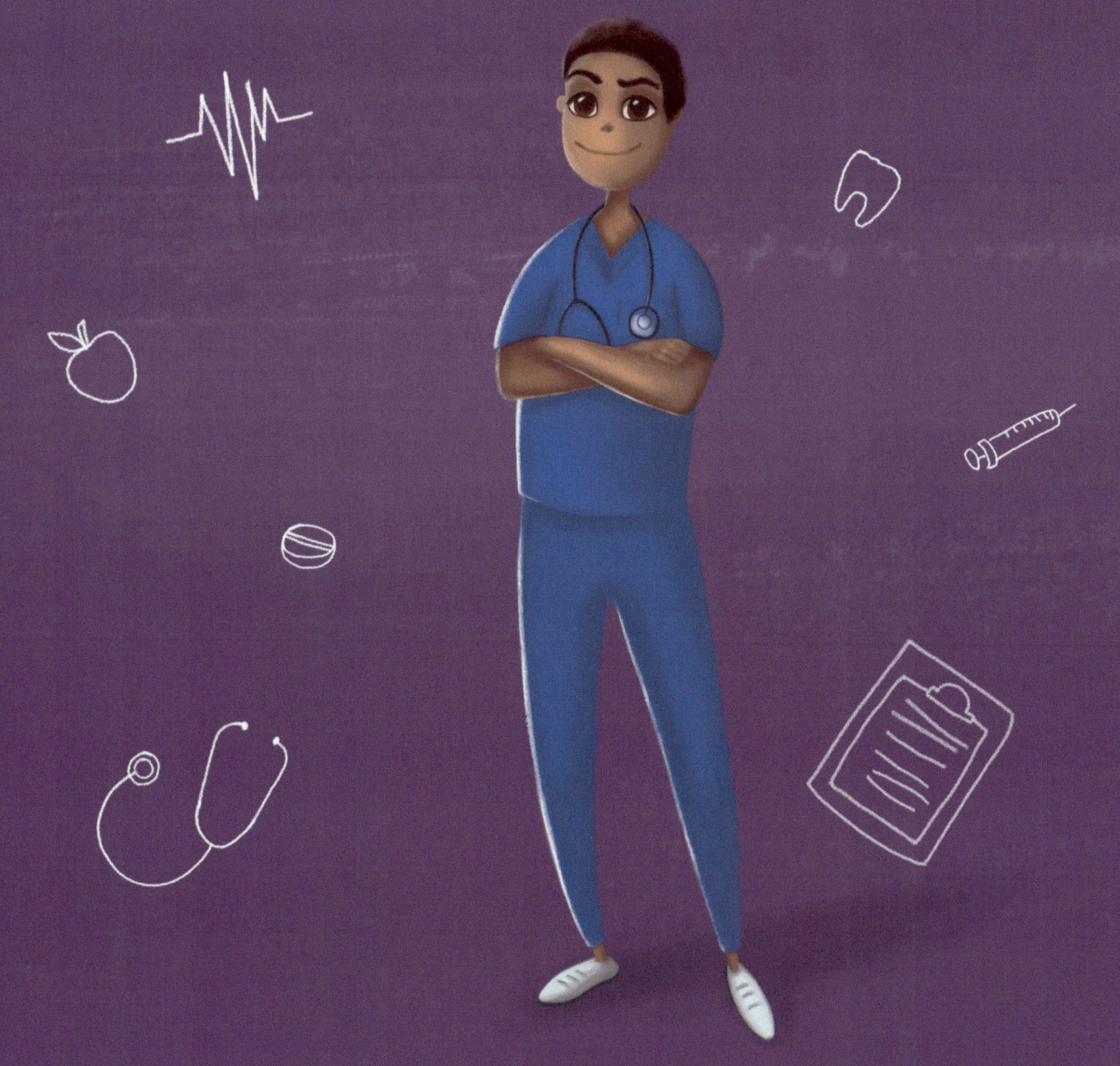

H is for Humble

Life as a nurse is filled with good and bad. Patients will praise the nurse for their dedication and caring. Despite the praise, the nurse remains humble, realizing they are the tool, the patient is the focus.

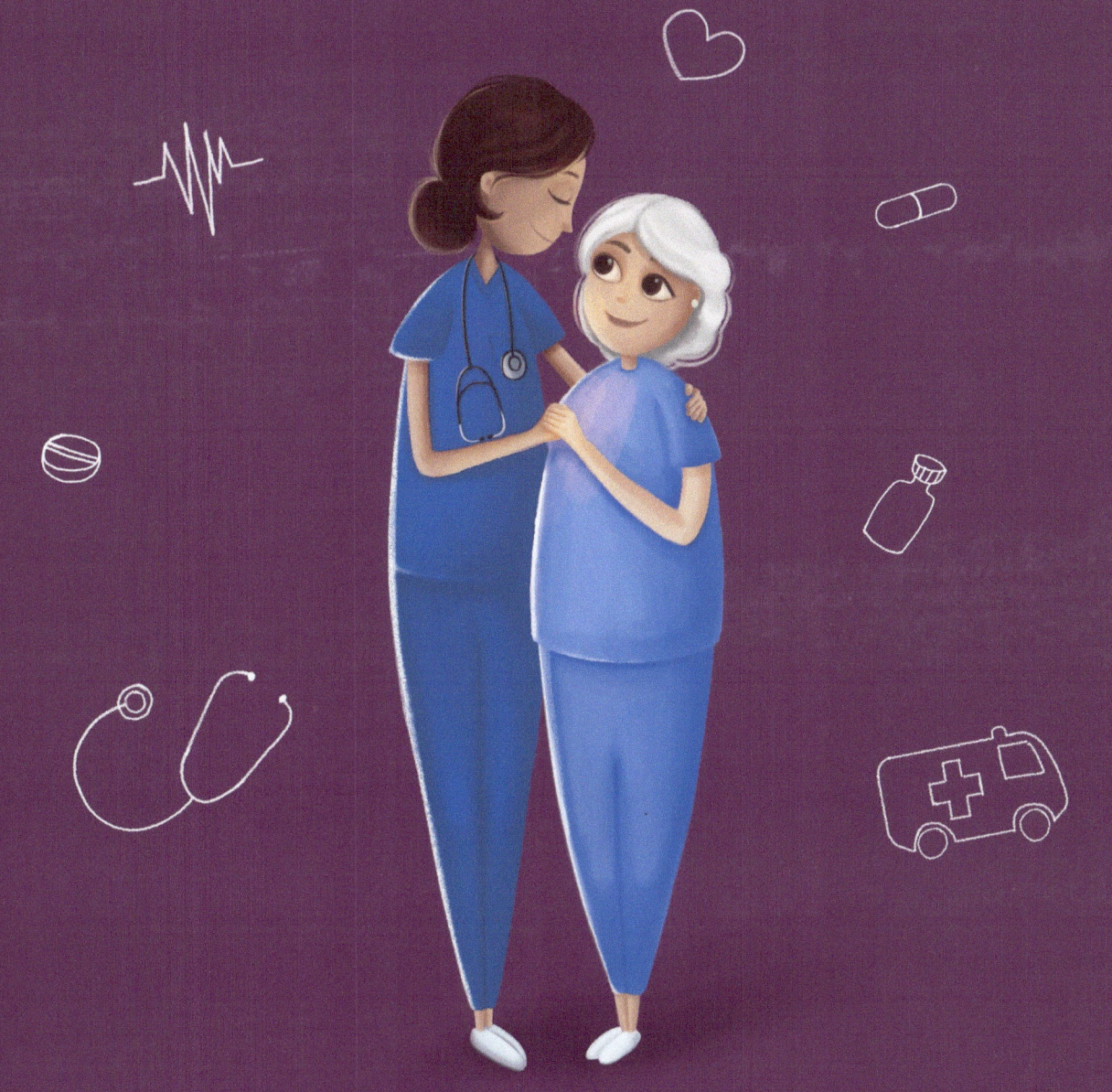

I

is for Irreplaceable

Nurses are the heart of healthcare. There is no replacement for the knowledge, skill, and duties of a nurse. The nurse bundles a million unique skills into one job . . . "nurse".

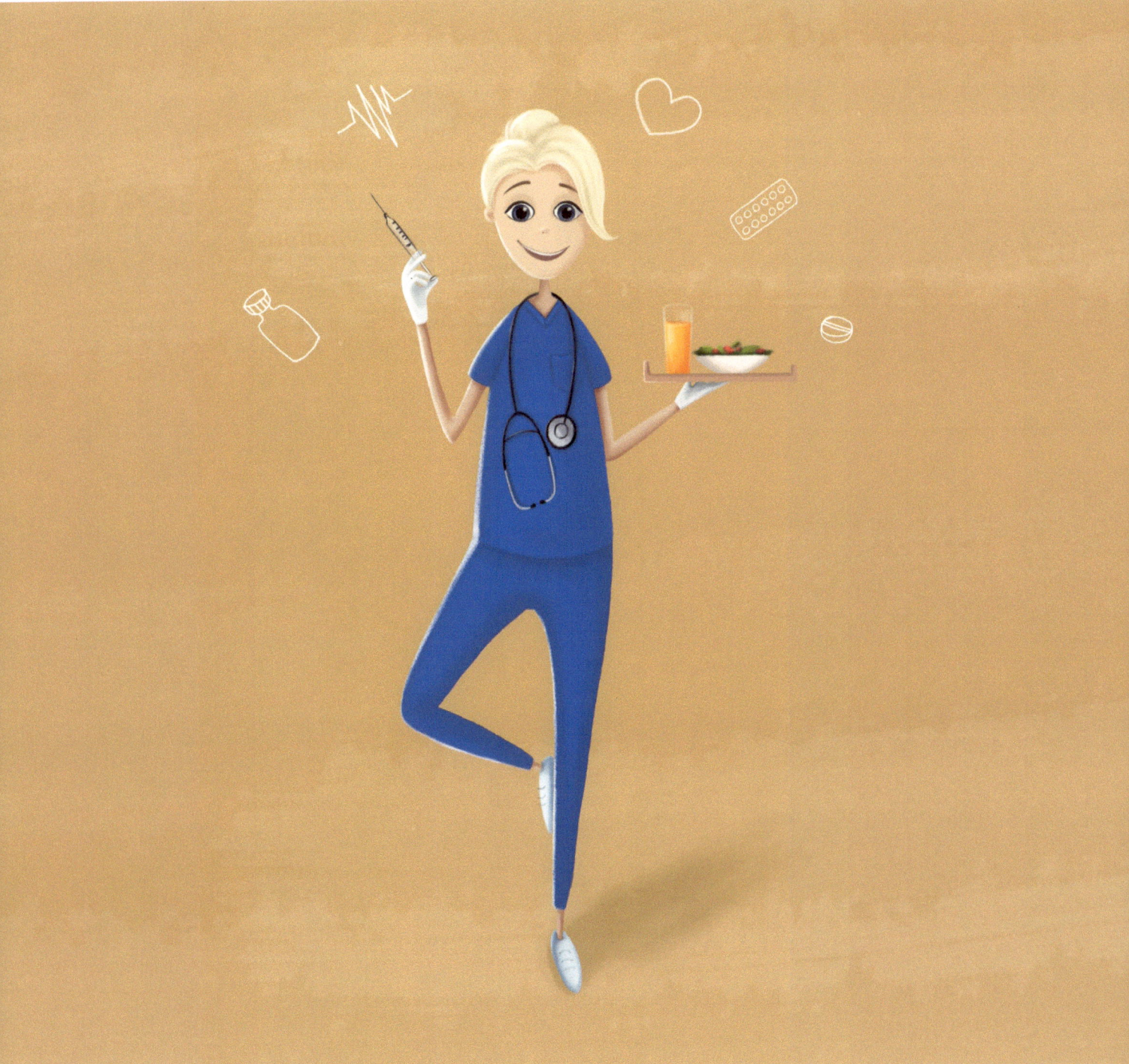

J

is for Joyful

The nurse will see death and heartache. The nurse will see the worst of the human condition. Through all this, the nurse remains joyful because their work fills the soul with a sense of purpose everyday.

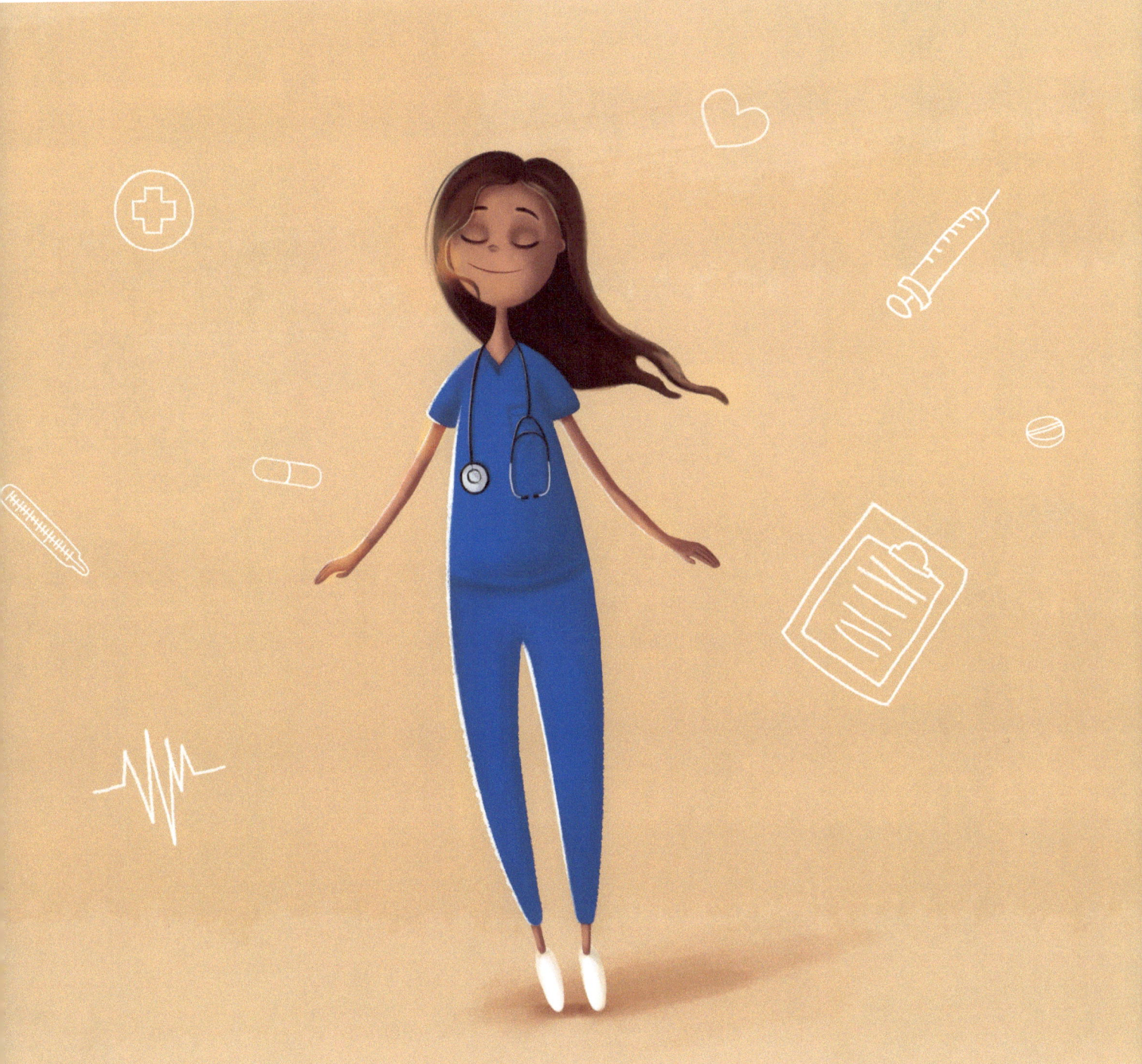

K is for Knowledgeable

Kindness helps, but without a deep knowledge, the nurse is unable to provide holistic care. The nurse has a voracious appetite for learning and growing.

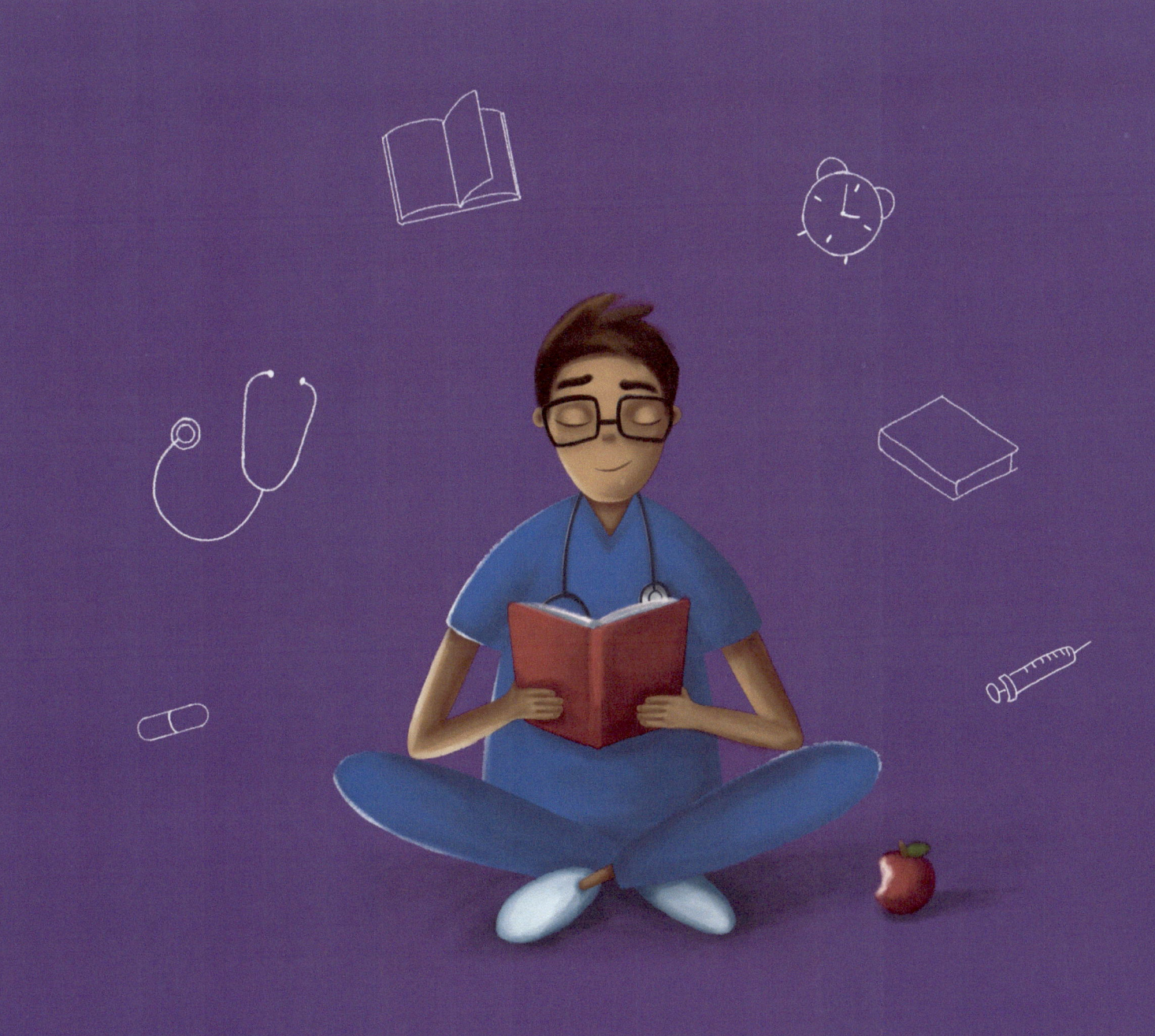

L

is for Loving

Nurses are filled with love. Love for life. Love for others.

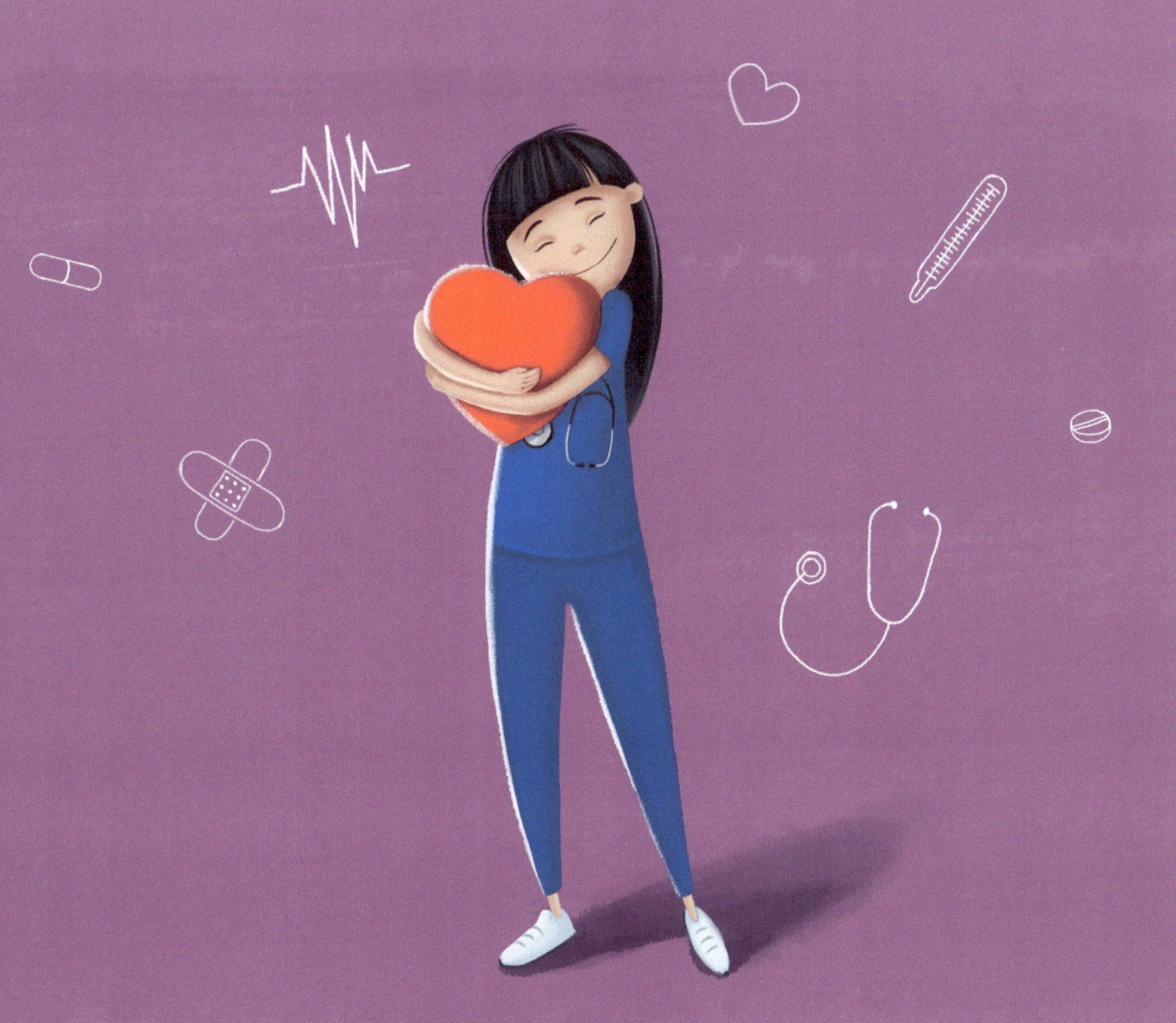

M is for Mindful

Sound decisions are made with deep thought. Throughout training, the nurse has learned to think. Nurses are comfortable contemplating and analyzing to determine the best option in complex situations.

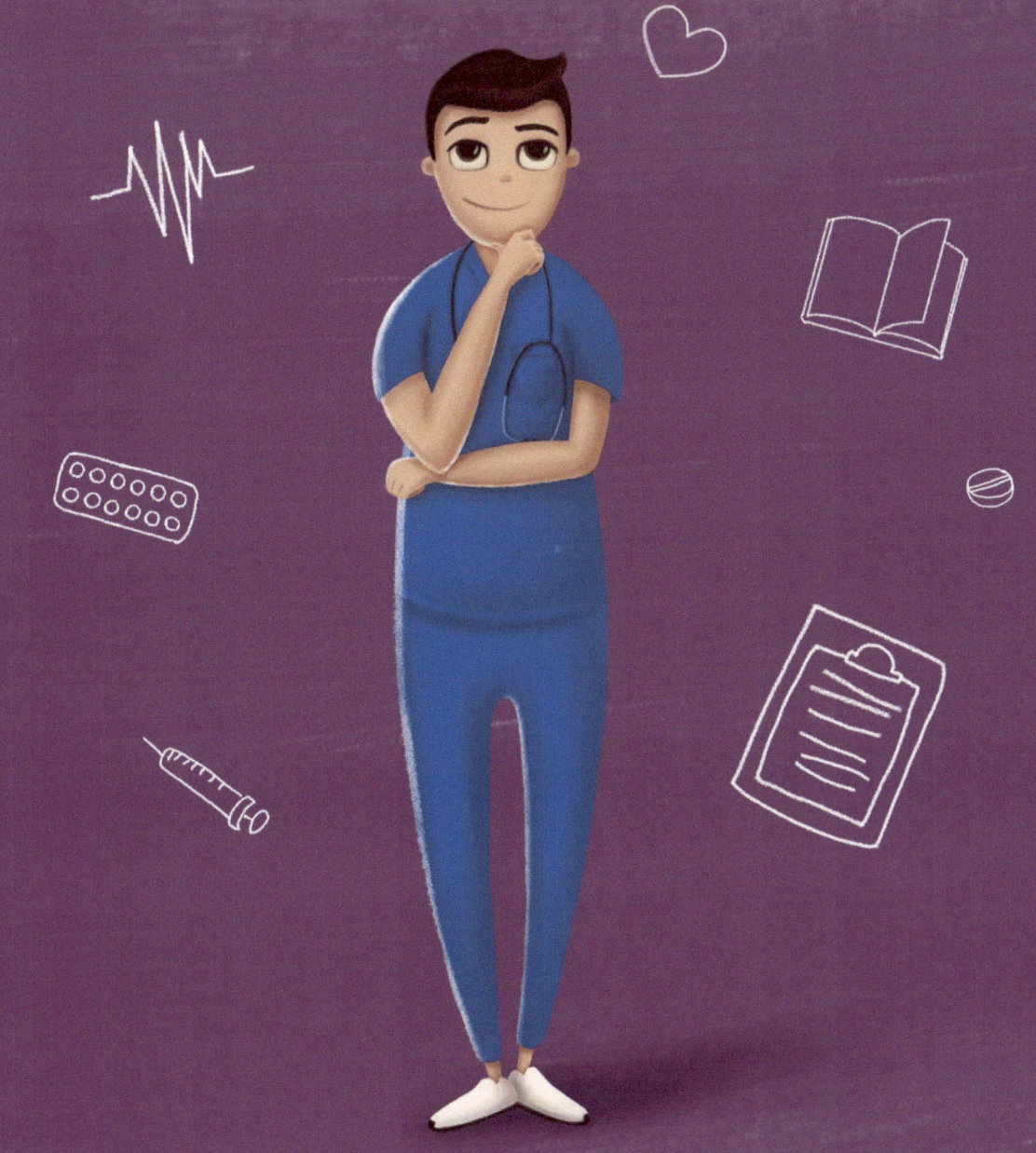

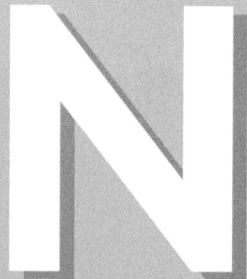 **is for Nurse**

Nurses are millions strong. Nurses are connected. When nurses meet, they "get it". No other job brings more purpose or meaning to life than Nurse.

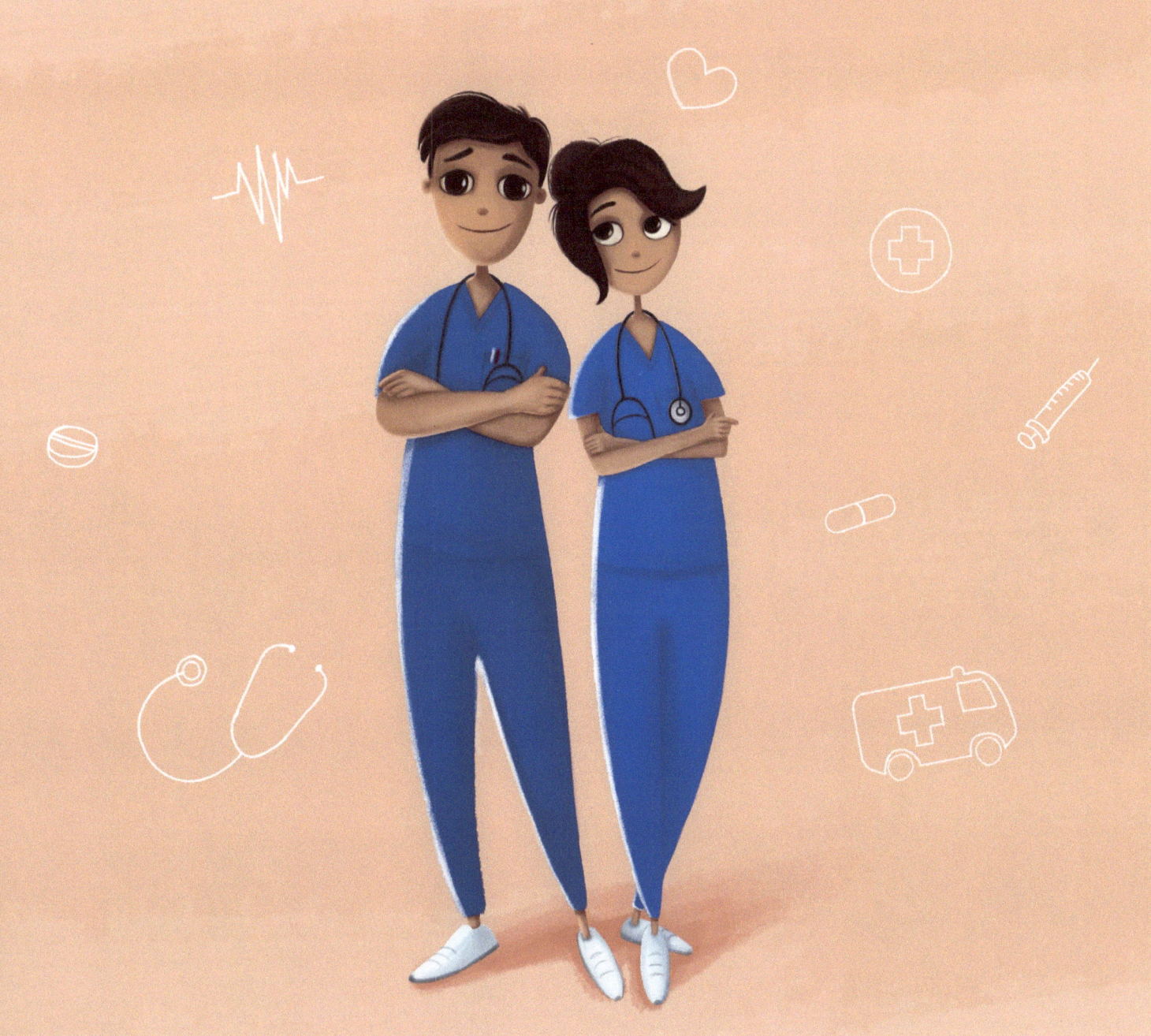

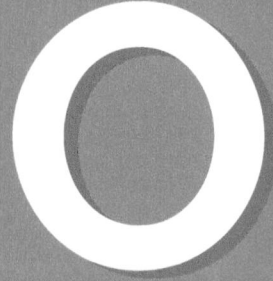

is for Organized

Managing multiple patients with different disease processes, different medications, different providers, different dynamics, different procedures, and different needs takes superhuman organization. The nurse makes this all look easy.

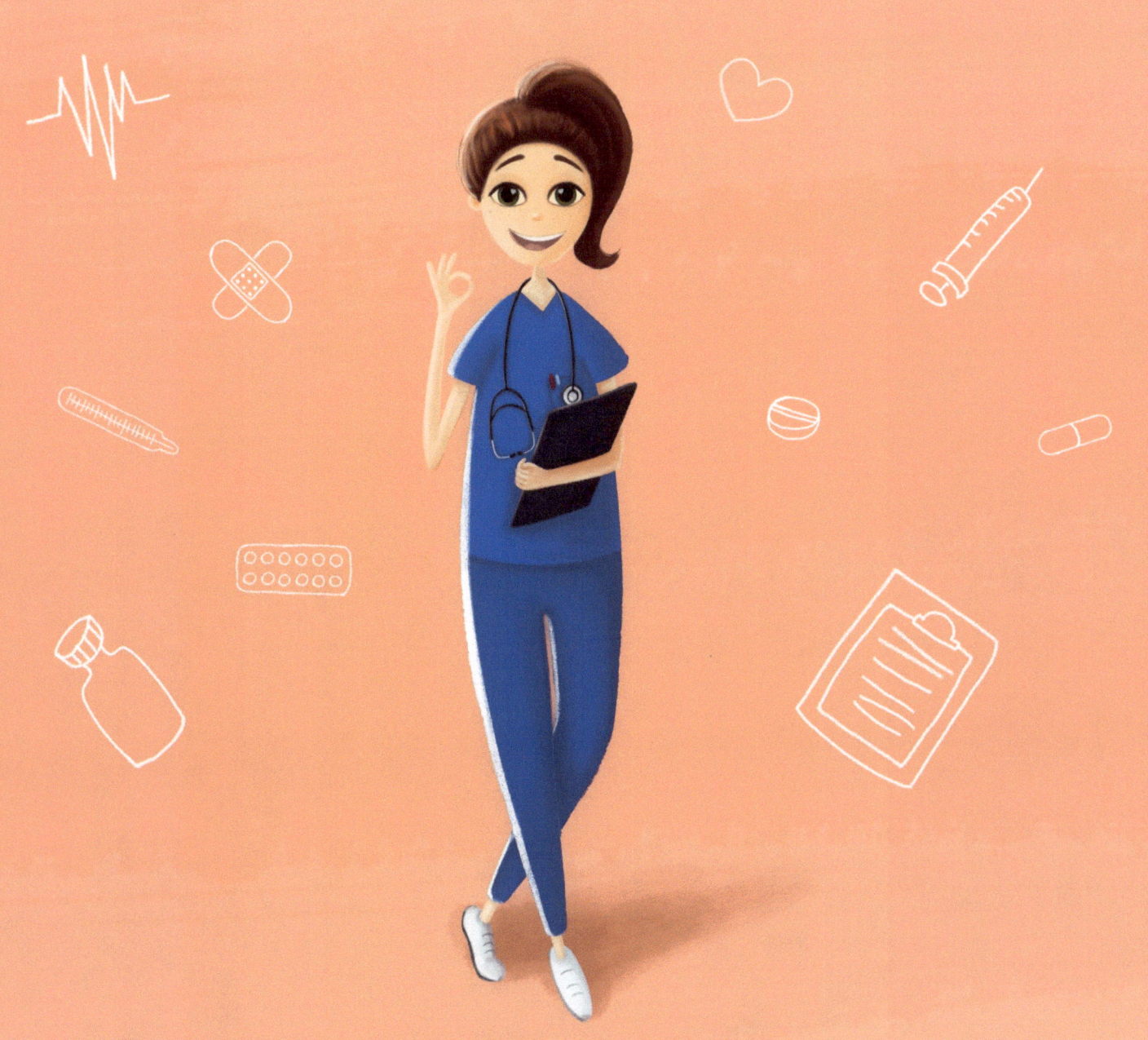

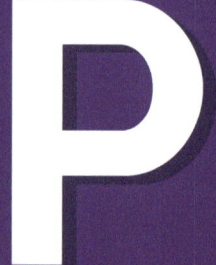

P

is for Patient

Lunch break might not be now, the transfer might not arrive now, the Doctor might not call back now, the meds might not arrive now. The nurse is patient. The nurse has learned to wait.

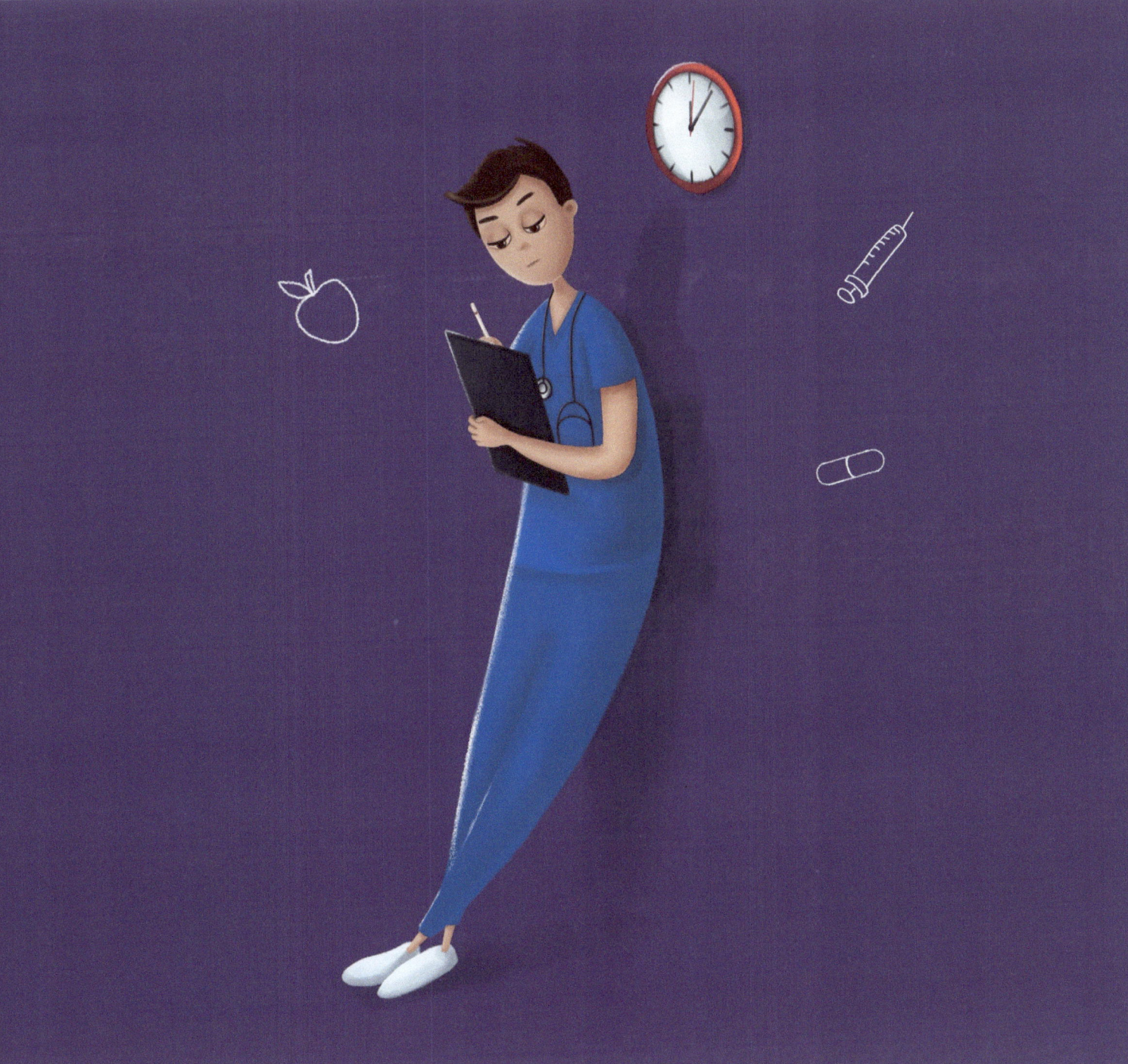

Q is for Quiet

The nurse knows when silence is the best response.

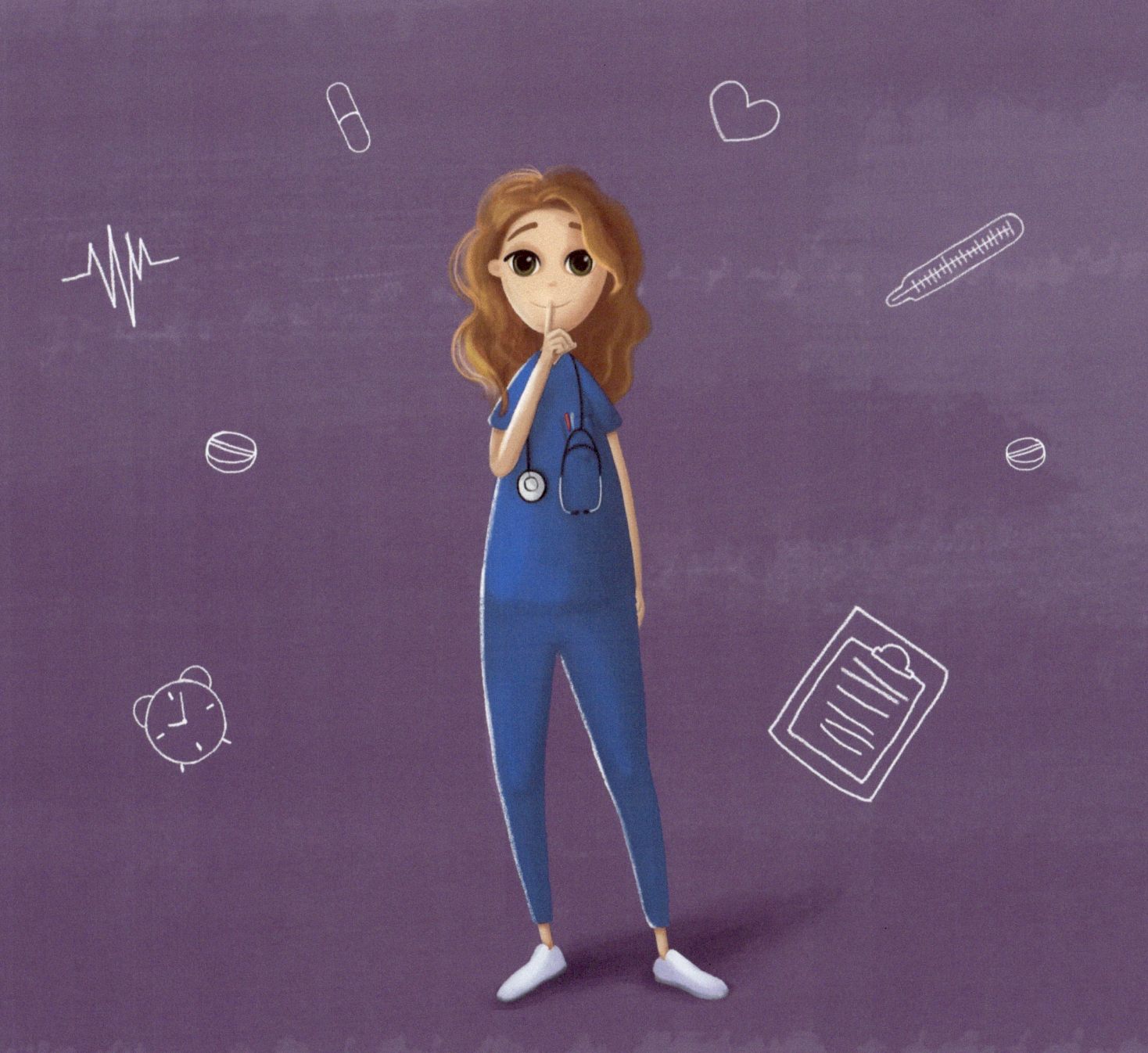

R

is for Respectful

The nurse will be kicked, hit, spit on, sworn at, and disrespected. In all this, the nurse has learned to respond with dignity and respect. The nurse knows how and when to respond.

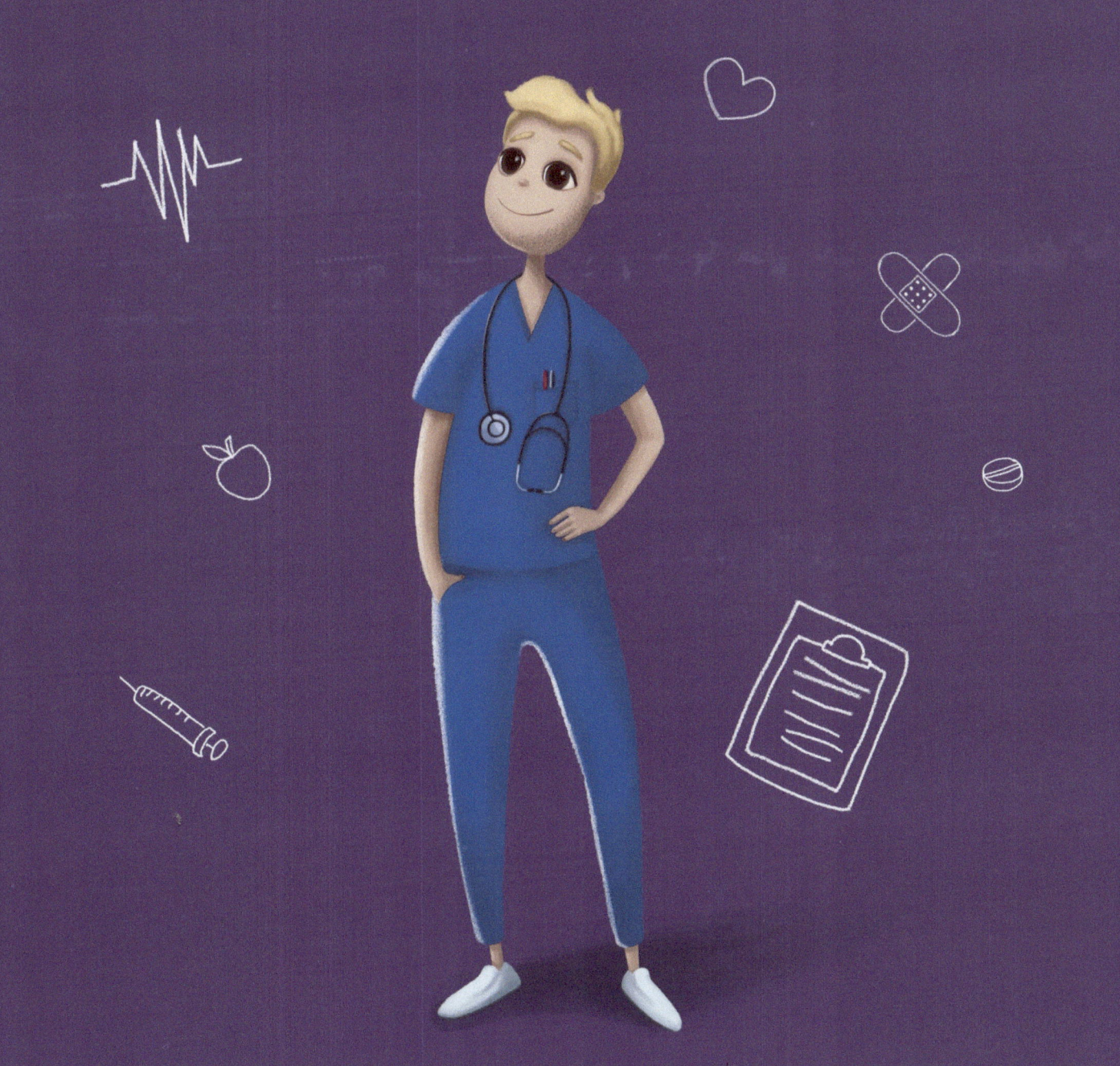

S

is for Selfless

From Florence until today, nurses know they will be giving of themselves every hour of every shift. They know that nursing is not self fulfilling. The nurse enters the field prepared to give and give and give.

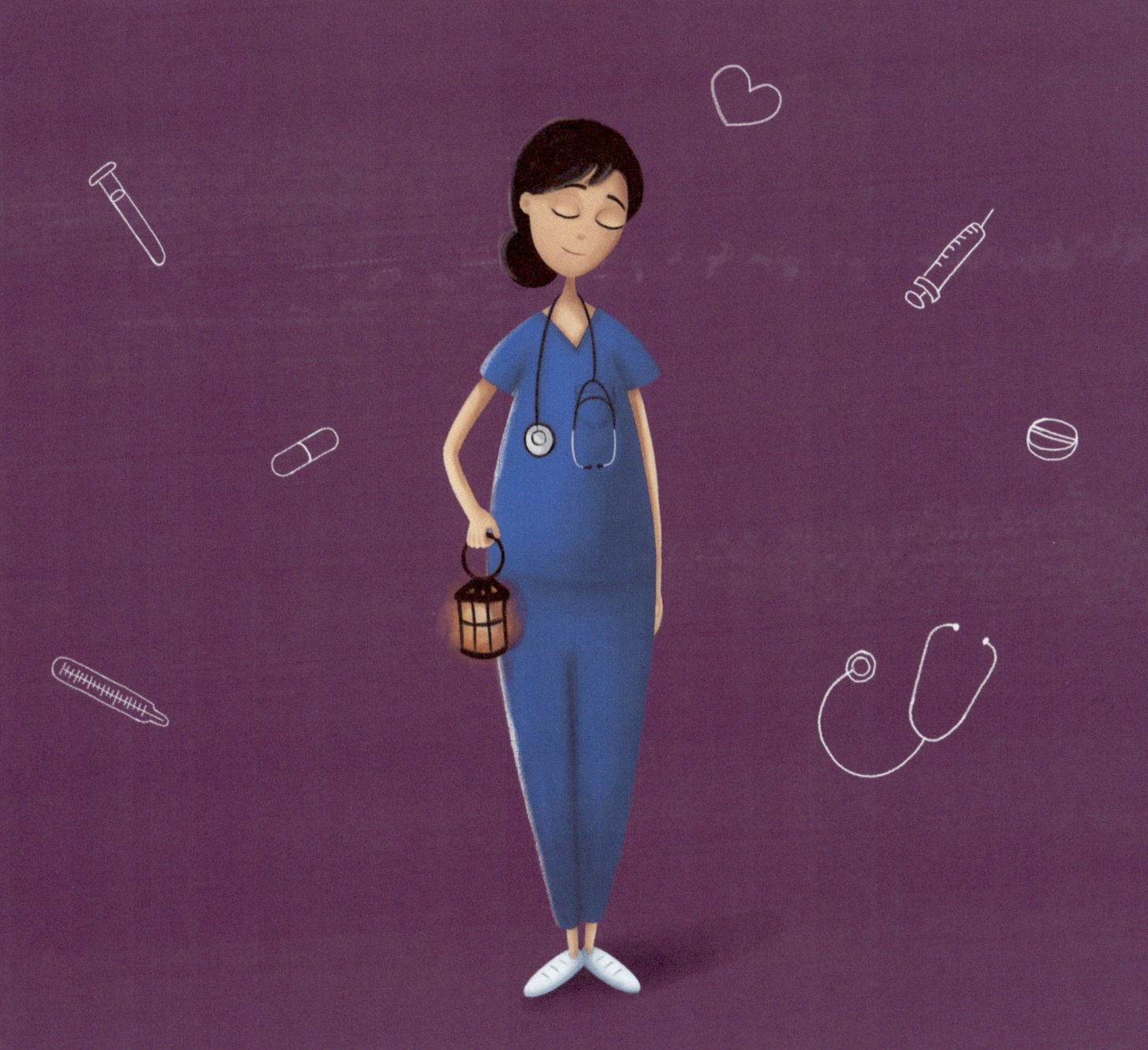

T

is for Teacher

Sharing the knowledge is one of the joys of nursing. Explaining to patients in a way they understand and become enabled makes the nurse a teacher every shift. If a nurse cares for 3 patients per shift and works for 25 years, they will teach 11,250 individuals. Every moment is a teaching moment.

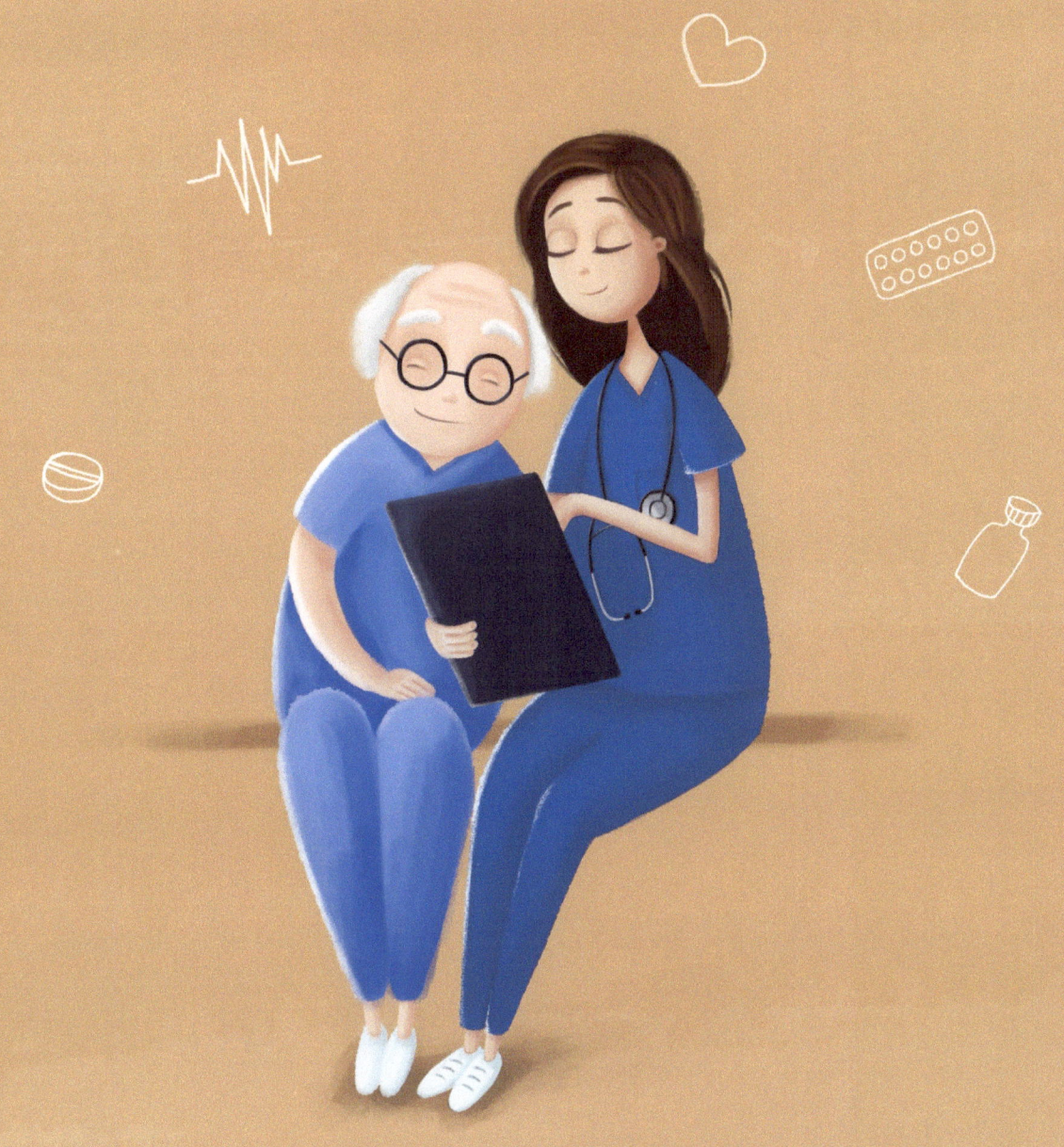

U

is for Understanding

A unique skill in modern times, the nurse is understanding of all. The nurse does not judge, the nurse does not discriminate. The nurse believes all deserve equal care and compassion.

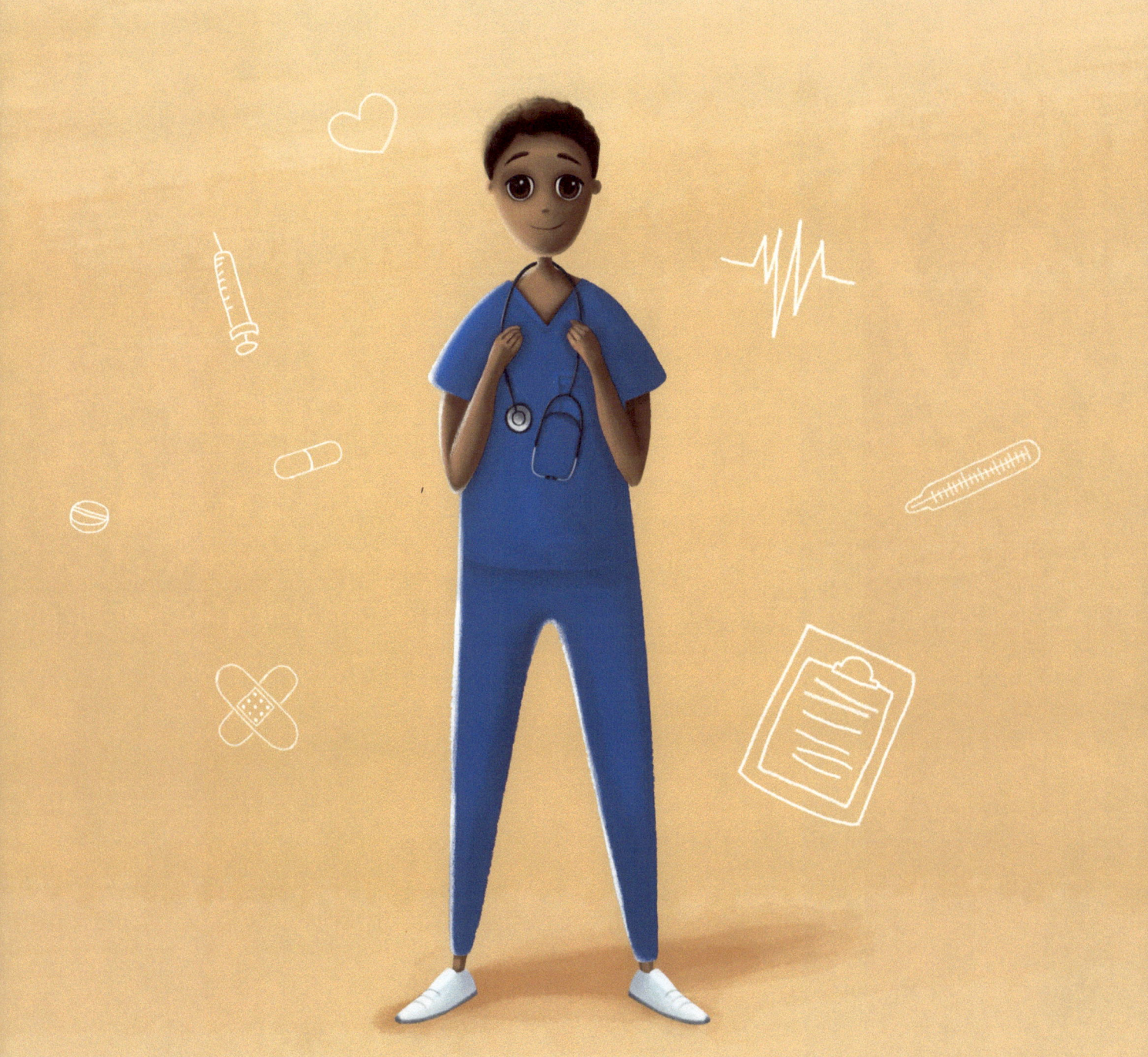

V

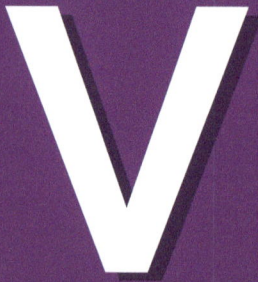

is for Veracious

The nurse is always learning, growing, improving. The nurse does not accept passive learning but has an appetite for chasing new knowledge and growth.

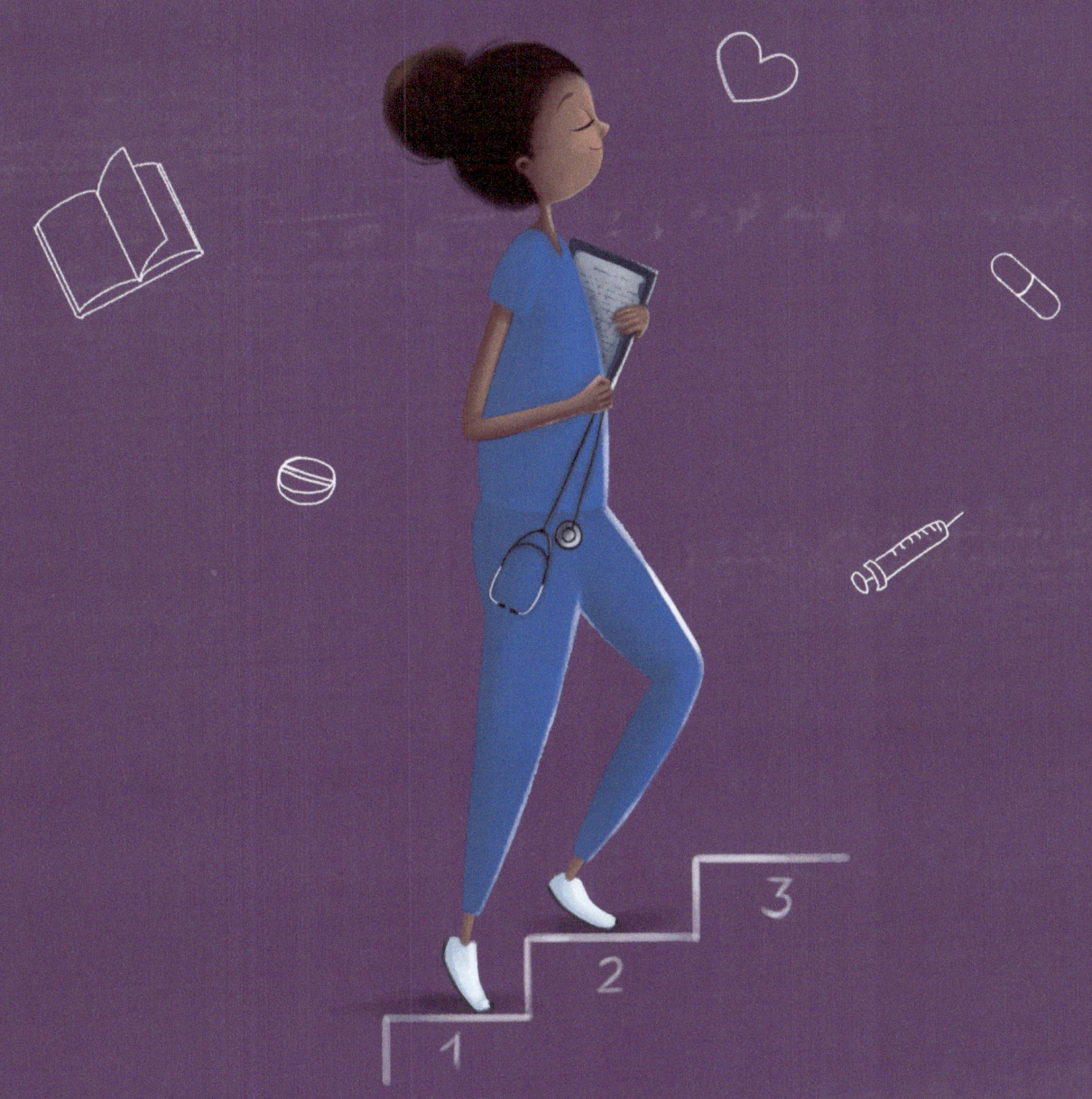

W is for Wise

In every decision, the nurse applies their knowledge, experience, and good judgement to make wise decisions. The nurse is pensive to avoid emotional decisions and thoughtful to consider all options.

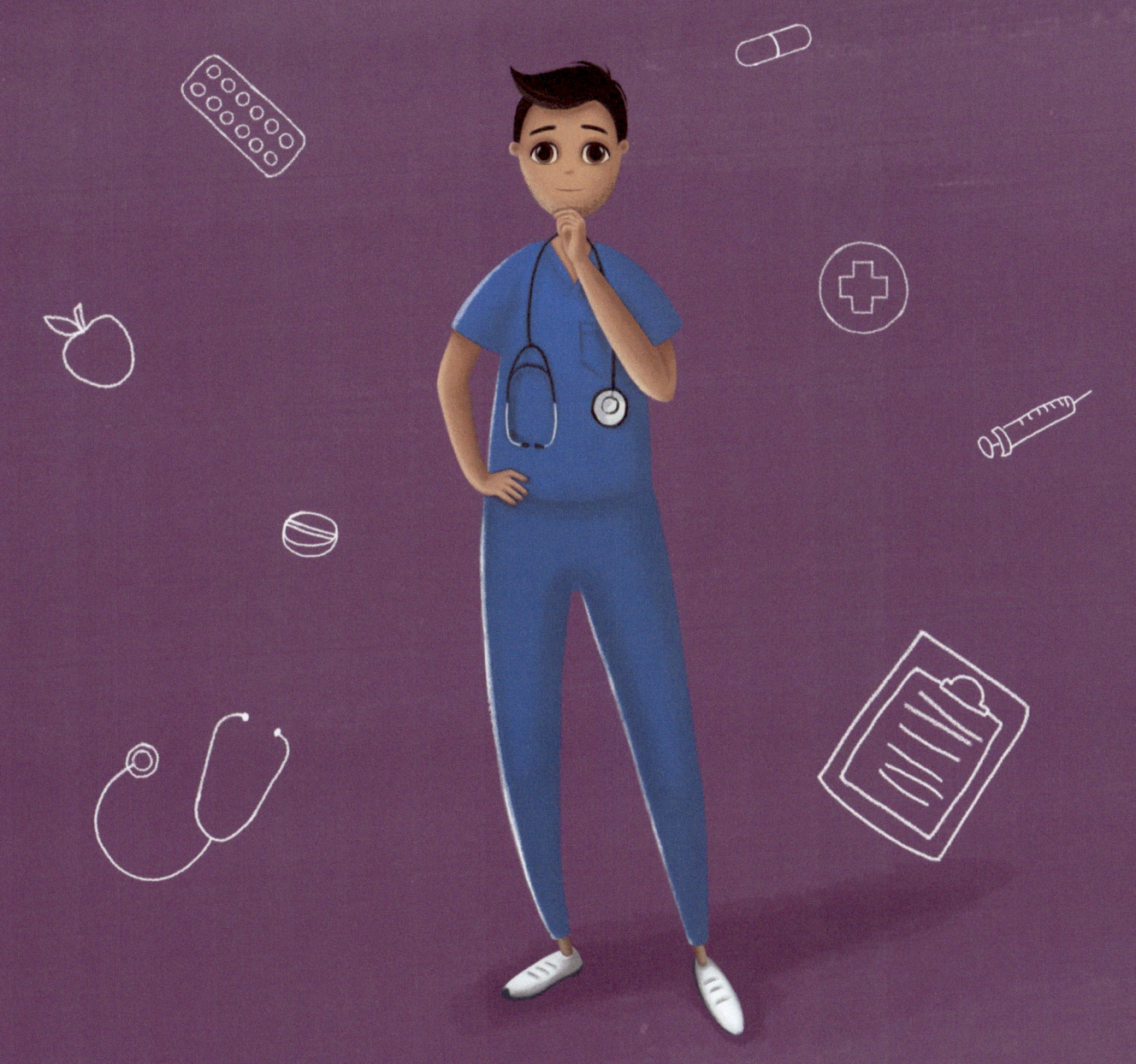

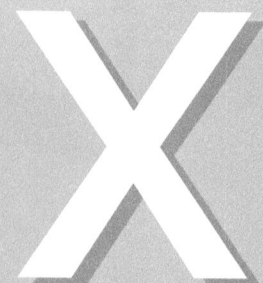

X is for Xanax

Sometimes, Xanax is the answer.

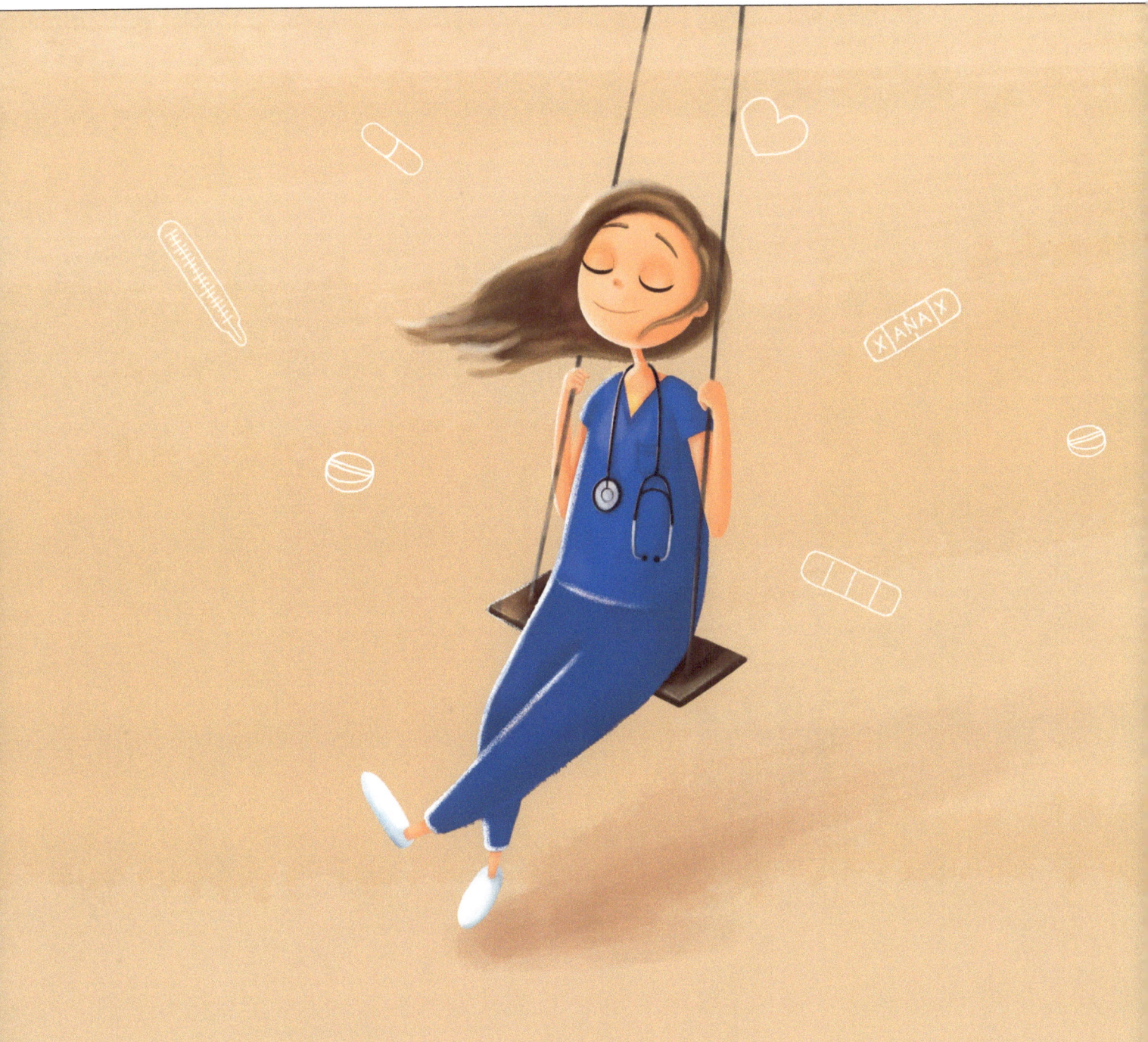

Y

is for Youthful

As the years roll on, the nurse stays young. Though the nurse will find a grey hair or two, gain a few pounds, and slow down a step, their soul remains young.

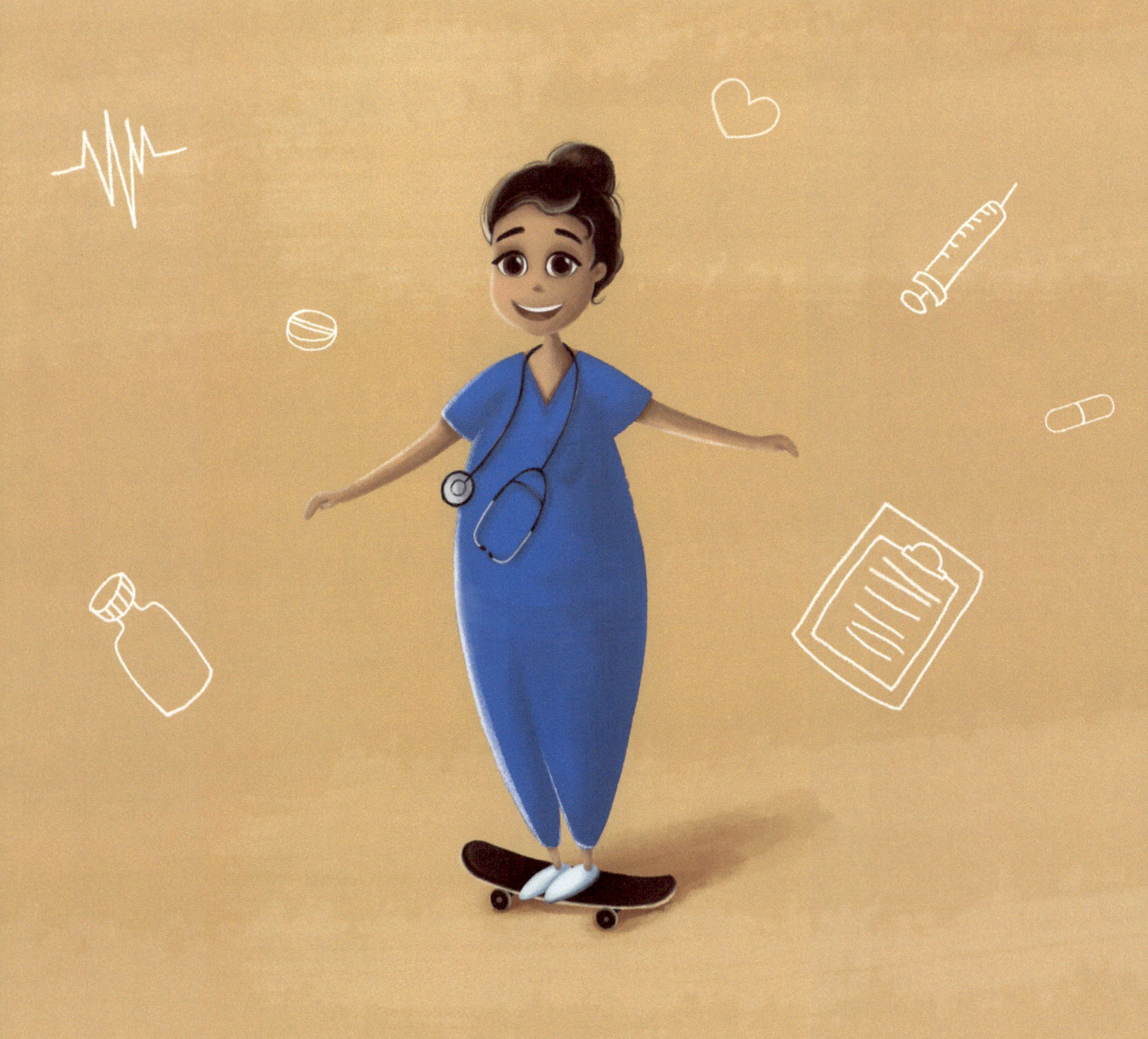

Z

is for Zealous

When it comes to caring for patients, the nurse has a relentless enthusiasm. Nursing requires superhuman focus and effort.

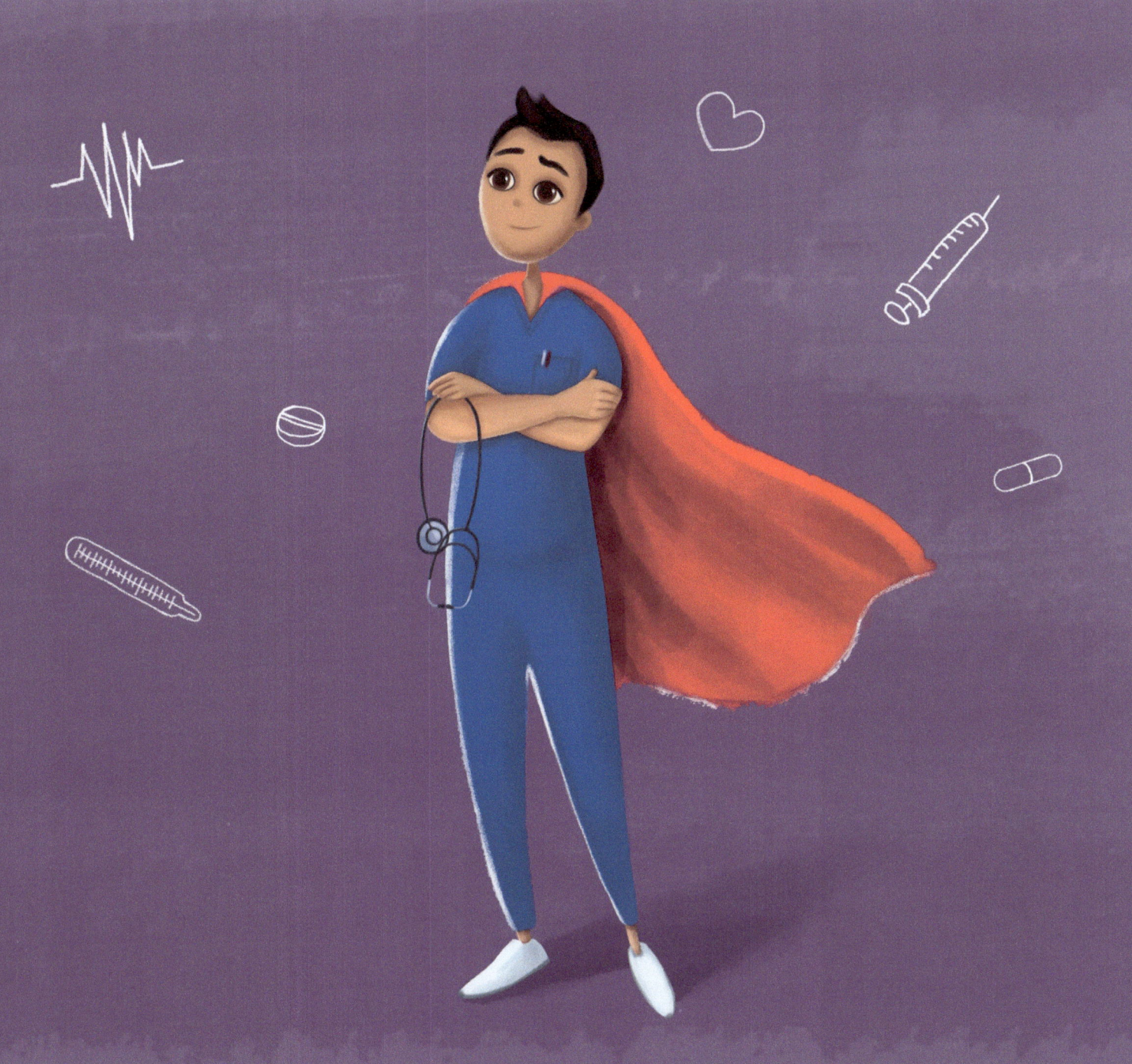

Being a nurse is more than a career.
Being a nurse is a calling.

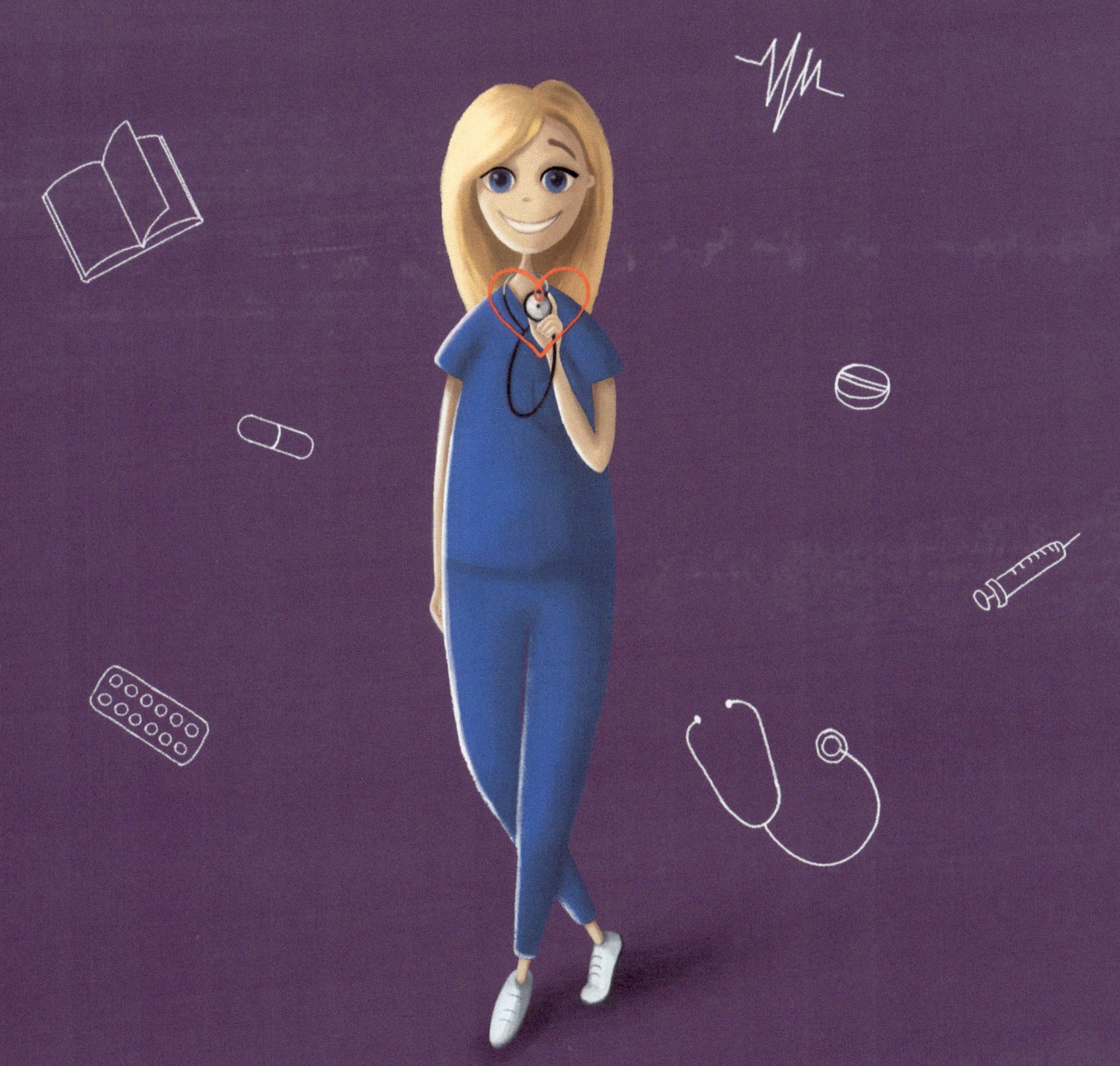

Nursing is more than a job. Nursing is who we are. Every fiber, every muscle, every beat of our hearts.

One big happy nursing family.
Healing patients happily.

It's something we feel deep within.
Proud to be RN.

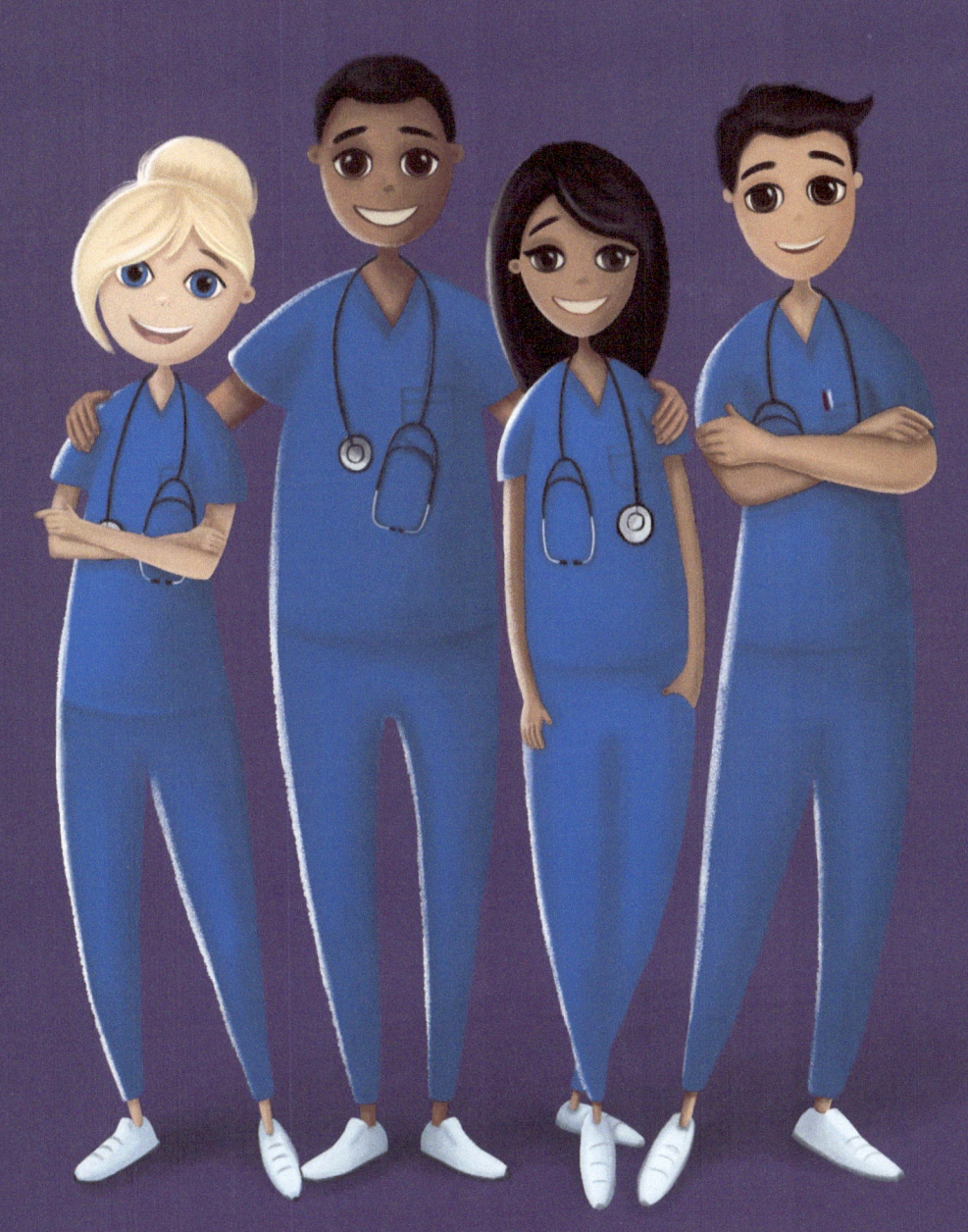

About the Author

Jon Haws RN BSN CCRN is a passionate nurse mentor and founder of NRSNG.com. Jon has worked in ICU/Trauma as a bedside nurse, preceptor, charge nurse, and code team nurse. In 2014, Jon founded NRSNG.com to provide tools and confidence to nursing students struggling through the education process.

www.ingramcontent.com/pod-product-compliance
Lightning Source LLC
Chambersburg PA
CBHW051048180526
45172CB00002B/558

* 9 7 8 1 5 4 8 3 0 9 2 9 9 *